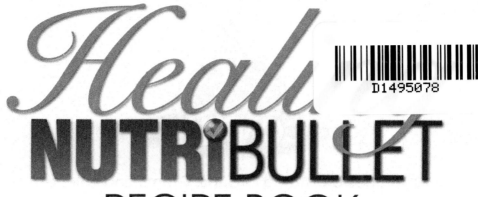

Healing NUTRiBULLET
RECIPE BOOK
200 Health Boosting Delicious and Optimally Nutritious Blast and Smoothie Recipes

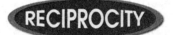

First Edition published by Reciprocity in 2014
All rights reserved

EDITOR
James Watkins

WRITERS
Marco Black
Oliver Lahoud

ILLUSTRATOR
David Joyce

NUTRITION ADVISOR
Sibel Osman

Disclaimer
The information in this book is provided on the basis that neither the authors nor the editors nor the publishers shall have any responsibility for any loss or damage that results or is claimed to have resulted from reading it. Some of the recipes contain nuts or nut milk. If you have a nut allergy please avoid those particular recipes.

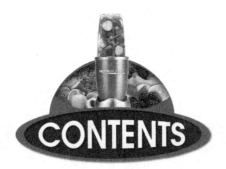

CONTENTS

All recipes are stated in Cups, Grams and Ounces.

*All recipes are stated in Cups, Grams and Ounces.
The precise nutritional break down into Protein grams, Fat grams, Carb
grams, Fibre grams and Kcals is calculated for each recipe using
data from the U.S. Department of Agriculture database.*

Health Benefits 9
Essential Amino Acids 10
Essential Vitamins 12
Essential Oils and Fats 12
Essential Minerals 13
Superfoods 13
Sleep and foods 16
Eat a Rainbow of Colour 18
Nutrition Data 19
NutriBullet Capacities 20
Cleaning and Warnings 20
Tips and Extras 22

Superfood Blasts
Made entirely out of Superfoods

Spinach Royale 24
Papaya goes Blueberry 24
Broccoli in Avocado 25
Broccoli kisses Chard 25
Chard invites Goji 26
Papaya and Flax Salad 26
Broccoli befriends Pumpkin 27
Chard Paradise 27
Broccoli partners Blueberry 28
Blueberry joins Flax 28
Chia Orchard 29

Guava Blend 29
Tomato Soother 30
Broccoli Sunshine 30
Flax Supermodel 31
Blueberry Explosion 31
Broccoli hugs Apricot 32
Beetroot Delivered 32
Chard Twist 33
Goji kisses Flax 33

Superfood Smoothies
Made entirely out of Superfoods

Blackberry and Goji Potion 34
Broccoli in Spinach 34
Papaya Delivered 35
Avocado Seduction 35
Broccoli Concerto 36
Papaya hugs Guava 36
Raspberry Dictator 37
Blueberry embraces Goji 37
Apricot Chorus 38
Chard and Guava Infusion 38
Blueberry hugs Beetroot 39
Spinach Treat 39
Carrot Opera 40
Spinach partners Avocado 40
Broccoli and Guava Explosion 41
Broccoli Soother 41
Chard and Blackberry Dream 42
Papaya Extravaganza 42
Broccoli and Goji Supermodel 43
Blackberry Fantasy 43

Anti Oxidizing Blasts
All ingredients are high in antioxidants

Green Cabbage hugs Broccoli 44
Red Cabbage goes Cranberry 44
Strawberry Wonder 45
Blackberry and Walnut Utopia 45
Papaya embraces Pecan 46

Broccoli Opera 46
Red Cabbage and Apple Surprise 47
Raspberry joins Sunflower 47
Pear meets Sesame 48
Cherry Heaven 48
Apple befriends Flax 49
Papaya Concerto 49
Red Cabbage and Cranberry Sunshine 50
Goji Delivered 50
Blueberry Miracle 51

Anti Oxidizing Smoothies
All ingredients are high in antioxidants

Spinach and Cherry Morning 51
Papaya Opera 52
Spinach Invigorator 52
Blueberry Ensemble 53
Prune Symphony 53

Detoxing and Cleansing Blasts
All ingredients have detoxing capabilities

Pineapple goes Sesame 54
Green Cabbage and Apple Vision 54
Watercress embraces Apple 55
Brazil Salad 55
Avocado hugs Grapefruit 56
Watercress meets Brazil 56
Broccoli Cocktail 57
Watercress and Apple Kiss 57
Green Cabbage and Grapefruit Mist 58
Fennel joins Apple 58
Fennel and Pineapple Blockbuster 59
Avocado Fiesta 59

Detoxing and Cleansing Smoothies
All ingredients have detoxing capabilities

Avocado partners Pineapple 60
Red Cabbage meets Apple 60

Green Cabbage and Apple Sonata 61
Watercress goes Apple 61
Watercress Mist 62
Fennel and Red Cabbage Dance 62
Broccoli Royale 63
Broccoli kisses Green Cabbage 63

Heart Care Blasts
Anti-inflammatory, high in Omega 3, anti oxidants, Vitamins C, E

Broccoli and Rocket Tonic 64
Lettuce and Orange Booster 64
Blueberry and Walnut Blend 65
Lettuce and Sesame Medley 65
Spinach befriends Blackberry 66
Orange and Pecan Salad 66
Raspberry Journey 67
Nectarine Blossom 67
Strawberry and Sesame Melody 68
Strawberry and Chia Soother 68
Tomato Vortex 69
Sesame Bonanza 69
Pecan Seduction 70
Nectarine and Cauliflower Delivered 70
Lettuce Fiesta 71
Red Pepper Paradise 71
Raspberry meets Cauliflower 72
Spinach Orchard 72
Broccoli befriends Chia 73
Raspberry Heaven 73

Blasts for Deeper Longer Sleep and Happiness
High in Tryptophan, Magnesium, Vitamins B3, B6, B9

Beetroot Sensation 74
Prune kisses Pumpkin 74
Watercress Fiesta 75
Apricot befriends Sunflower 75
Prune and Beetroot Sunrise 76
Spinach Royale 76
Watercress and Apricot Tango 77
Prune embraces Carrot 77

Broccoli Morning 78
Spinach invites Watercress 78
Fine Bean Dance 79
Pumpkin Delusion 79
Avocado in Cashew 80
Prune Embrace 80
Apricot Blend 81
Watercress and Broccoli Constellation 81
Carrot Consortium 82
Broccoli meets Prune 82
Sesame Mirage 83
Apricot and Cashew Contradiction 83

Clear Thinking Brain Food Blasts
High in Omega3, Beta Carotene, Lycopene, Magnesium, Zinc, Vitamins B, C, E

Strawberry goes Walnut 84
Rocket partners Pumpkin 84
Blueberry and Brazil Morning 85
Blackberry Booster 85
Rocket and Strawberry Fandango 86
Bok Choy and Avocado Melody 86
Hazelnut Debut 87
Green Cabbage Delight 87
Rocket and Blueberry Journey 88
Blueberry and Almond Royale 88
Strawberry Heaven 89
Watercress and Strawberry Orchard 89
Spinach Kiss 90
Mint embraces Strawberry 90
Green Cabbage and Mint Ensemble 91
Cashew Elixir 91
Green Cabbage and Bok Choy Panacea 92
Mint goes Rocket 92
Watercress Galaxy 93
Blueberry Cornucopia 93

Radiant Skin Nourishing Blasts
High in Anti oxidants, Caroteinoids, Polyphenols, Pectin, Zinc, Vitamins A, C

Mint joins Raspberry 94
Mint and Pumpkin Dictator 94
Watercress invites Nectarine 95

Apple befriends Red Grape 95
Rocket Mirage 96
Watercress and Pecan Embrace 96
Cranberry embraces Cashew 97
Green Cabbage and Blackberry Presented 97
Cashew Galaxy 98
Sesame Twist 98
Goji and Pecan Machine 99
Nectarine goes Pumpkin 99
Watercress hugs Pecan 100
Pumpkin Vision 100
Prune Dance 101
Plum in Cashew 101
Rocket and Watercress Soother 102
Mint kisses Spinach 102
Bok Choy and Red Grape Blossom 103
Green Cabbage partners Pecan 103

Immunity Boosting Blasts
*Supergreens and foods high in Carotenoids, Sulphoraphane,
Indoles, Fibre, Selenium, Vitamins C, D3, E*

Flax Delusion 104
Spinach and Broccoli Paradox 104
Green Cabbage and Chia Consortium 105
Apricot and Carrot Vision 105
Spinach meets Broccoli 106
Strawberry kisses Yellow Pepper 106
Red Pepper Mirage 107
Orange embraces Flax 107
Grapefruit and Carrot Salad 108
Mango hugs Flax 108
Papaya and Red Pepper Sunshine 109
Green Cabbage Fantasy 109
Broccoli Delivered 110
Tangerine Royale 110
Carrot Waterfall 111
Green Cabbage befriends Brazil 111
Green Cabbage and Spinach Cornucopia .112
Red Grape in Brazil 112
Broccoli joins Apricot 113
Apricot partners Flax 113

Immunity Boosting Smoothies
Supergreens and foods high in Carotenoids, Sulphoraphane, Indoles, Fibre, Selenium, Vitamins C, D3, E

Broccoli and Mango Garden 114
Apricot and Beetroot Fiesta 114
Spinach Tango 115
Tangerine and Tomato Mirage 115
Spinach partners Broccoli 116
Green Cabbage meets Strawberry 116
Beetroot Bonanza 117
Green Cabbage in Orange 117
Green Cabbage Sonata 118
Yellow Pepper Cornucopia 118
Apricot and Yellow Pepper Creation 119
Spinach and Broccoli Blend 119
Spinach and Tangerine Bliss 120
Broccoli embraces Blueberry 120
Papaya Machine 121
Carrot Feast 121
Green Cabbage and Strawberry Utopia 122
Orange Kiss 122
Apricot Revision 123
Papaya and Carrot Sunrise 123

Notes 124

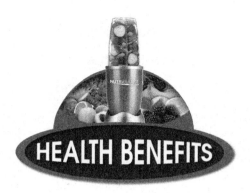

The Health Benefits of
NutriBullet Raw Vegetable Variation

Many clinical studies have shown that raw vegetables help fight the big killers today. They help significantly to fight Cancer (the more veggies and the less meat you eat the better your body can prevent and fight tumours). There was a wonderful study done on the Norwegians during the second world war when the German occupiers commandeered all their meat. The result was that the incidence of all types of cancer in Norwegians fell by more than 50%.

They help fight Cardio Vascular Disease. They provide essential antioxidants, oils, minerals, vitamins and are generally better for us than a hamburger or a pork sausage. But the trouble is that they normally do not taste as good as a hamburger or a pork sausage unless they are roasted with cheese or boiled to the point where they have lost most of their goodness.

This is where the NutriBullet comes in. It makes veggies taste great. A nutriblast can taste as good and as invigorating as a steak with fries or a cappuccino with a croissant or a chocolate torte with cream. Your mother would never have had to tell you to: "Eat your Greens" had your family possessed a NutriBullet.

The manufacturers claim all sorts of health benefits from it. And without going into medical detail, whatever the goodness is in a vegetable or leafy green or fruit or nut or seed, the NutriBullet can get that goodness out without destroying the delicate biochemical compounds with heat from cooking them. It is billed not as a blender or a juicer, but as an extractor. This is because the machine represents the best method mankind presently has of extracting the goodness from non meat food. The blades break down the cell walls of the ingredients and thereby release the cell contents into your intestines. So unless you have teeth which can rotate at 10,000 rpm, the NutriBullet represents a significant advance on chewing.

The other psychological trait of mankind which works against us here, is that we are loyal to what we like. Most of retail commerce is based upon brand loyalty. Although this type of loyalty doesn't always work so well with romantic partners! So we find a vegetable we like and then just eat that all the time. I mean once I have a record that I like, I will listen to it over and over again. So even if we do eat some vegetables or leafy greens or fruits, they will tend to be repetitions of a very small selection of what is available. They will just the ones that we have become familiar with and grown to like. They are essentially the vegetable next door.

So the purpose of this book is to empower to reader to vary their vegetables and fruits and greens and nuts and seeds on a daily basis. That is why we have included so many delicious Blasts and Smoothies. If you only drink a small fraction of these NutriBullet recipes you will be deficient in nothing that nature provides from Vegetables, Fruits, Nuts, Seeds and Greens.

Certain amino acids (protein) and fatty acids (fat) vitamins and minerals cannot be manufactured by the body. So they have to be eaten. This is one of the reasons why food variation is so important. Failing to eat certain essential foods can be lethal – even if you are putting on weight from all the food that you are eating! This was discovered when canned liquid diets were first invented. Some of the people who tried these out for more than a month just dropped dead due to running out of essential amino acids.

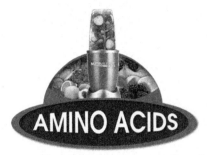

Essential Amino Acids

There are 11 of them: Tryptophan, Threonine, Isoleucine, Histidine Leucine, Lysine, Methionine + Cysteine, Phenylaneline + Tyrosine and Valine. These are nicely distributed throughout the leafy greens. Although meat and dairy have more protein and therefore more essential amino acids than greens per gram they have less protein than greens per kcal. So for dieters, Spinach (yummy) and Kale (fried in olive oil) are a good option.

Here are the Recommended Daily Intakes (RDI) or Recommended Daily Allowances (RDA) and Eastimated Average Requirements (EAR) for protein for 75kg/165lb men and for 64kg/140lb women.

Sex Age	EAR grams per day	RDI = RDA grams per day
165lb Men 19-30	52g	64g
165lb Men 30-50	52g	64g
165lb Men 50-70	52g	64g
165lb Men 70+	65g	81g
140lb Women 19-30	38g	48g
140lb Women 30-50	38g	48g

140lb Women 50-70	38g	48g
140lb Women 70+	48g	60g
140lb Pregnant Women	51g	64g
140lb Lactating Women	56g	70g

EAR is the estimated average requirement for 50% of people (i.e. for the average person) RDI/RDA is 20% higher and would work for 97% of the people. The figures are all linear so if you weight more then you should eat propoertionately more protein. RDI/RDA is 20% more than EAR.

The Essential Amino Acids should be eaten according to the following pattern in milligrams of essential amino acid per gram of protein intake...

Essential Amino Acid	RDI in mg per gram of Protein
Histidine	18mg
Isoleucine	25mg
Leucine	55mg
Lysine	51mg
Methionine + Cysteine	25mg
Phenylalanine + Tyrosine	47mg
Threonine	27mg
Tryptophan	7mg
Valine	32mg

So for a 75kg 50 year old man,with an RDI=RDA of 64grams of protein per day the Essential Amino Acid EARs are...

Essential Amino Acid	RDI in gram per day for a 64g perday Protein RDI
Histidine	1.15g
Isoleucine	1.64g
Leucine	3.52g
Lysine	3.26g
Methionine + Cysteine	1.60g
Phenylalanine + Tyrosine	3.01g
Threonine	1.73g
Tryptophan	0.45g
Valine	2.05g

One 200 ml glass of whole milk has between 24-42% of the Recommended Daily Intake of all of the 9 essential amino acid groups. We use 200 ml of whole milk in some of our Blast and Smoothie Recipes.

Protein powder (from milk) can be added to Smoothies to boost the protein content (Whey, Soy, Pea or Rice Protein powders are readily available). This may be necessary for men on a low calorie diet. Good whey protein power has around 76 grams of protein per 100 grams of the powder which provides around 378 kcal of energy.

Essential Amino Acid	Grams per 50 grams of Whey Protein Powder
Histidine	0.65g
Isoleucine	2.35g
Leucine	3.95g
Lysine	3.55g
Methionine + Cysteine	1.60g
Phenylalanine + Tyrosine	2.05g
Threonine	2.5g
Tryptophan	0.50g
Valine	2.20g

50 grams of Whey Protein Powder, although having only 38 grams of protein within it will provide the full RDI of all essential amino acids for a 50 year old 75kg man except in the cases of Phenylalanine+Tyrosine where it only provides 68% (2.05g) of the RDI (3.01g) and Histidine where it only provides 56% (0.65g) of the RDI (1.15g).

This is why body builders use whey protein shakes. But low calorie dieters can benefit from them too. Women can just add 20 grams of whey protein powder and men can add 30 grams to a Nutribullet recipe and half of your essential amino acid requirements are met instantly.

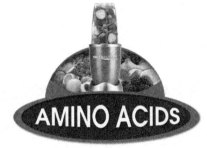

AMINO ACIDS

Essential Vitamins

These are: A, B1 (Thiamin), B2 (Riboflavin), B3 (Niacin), B4 (Choline/Adenine)) B5 (Pantotheic Acid), B6 (Pyridoxines), B7 (Biotin)B9 (Folates), B12 (Cobalamin), C, D3, E, K

Stop Press: The latest EU guidelines for Vitamin D3 are now 4000 IU per day rather than 400! Also the latest research shows that high dose Vitamin D3 toxicity is caused by a lack of Vitamin K2. Spinach and Kale are rich in K1 which the body can convert into K2. But 100 micrograms of K2 supplementation (MK7 variety) is recommended for each 1000 IU of Vitamin D3. Vitamin K2 is expensive so eat your dark leafy greens!

Essential Oils and Fats

This is a very short list. Basically the more fish based Omega3 (EPA DHA in particular) the better up to around 5 grams per day. And the more seed nut or vegetable based Omega3 (ALA) the better without limit.

There is plenty of evidence that Omega 3 in your diet has a large effect upon the cardio vascular system. In particular the Omega3 fish based or vegetable and seed based fatty acids should be eaten in larger amounts if you are on a high fat diet. There are good Omega3 supplements out there but whole foods containing Omega3 normally provide better absorption into the body than Omega3 supplements.

The 10 Essential Minerals

Calcium, Copper, Iron, Magnesium, Manganese, Phosphours, Potassium, Selenium, Sodium, Zinc

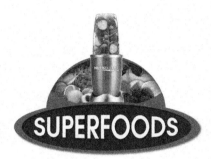

25 Widely Recognized Superfoods

These Superfoods contain many of the essential amino acids, fats, vitamins and minerals. But that is not why they are superfoods. They are defined as superfoods due to the health benefits that they confer. They are generally rich in anthocyanins, polyphenols, flavenoids, antioxidants, cancer fighting ellagic acid, heart disease fighting lycopene and other really useful nutrients which whilst not essential (in the sense that they can be manufactured by the body if it has the right components to hand), promote good health, fitness and well being. Between them these Superfoods are attributed with the following health benefits...

Increased Protection from Bacterial and Viral Infections
Increased Immune Function
Reduced Cancer Risk
Protection Against Heart Disease
Slowing Aging
DNA Repair and Protection
Prevention and reduction of Cardiovascular Disease
Reduced Hypertension (High Blood Pressure)
Alzheimer's Protection
Osteoporosis Protection
Stroke Prevention
Reduced Risk of Colon Cancer

Protection Against Heart Disease
Antioxidant Protection
Prevention of Epileptic Seizures
Prevention of Alopecia (Spot Baldness)
Reduced Risk of Type II Diabetes
Reduced Frequency of Migraine Headaches
Alleviation of Premenstrual Syndrome (PMS)
Regulation of Blood Sugar and Insulin Dependence
Slowing the progression of AIDS
Protection Against Dementia
Improved Eye Health
Alleviation of Inflammation
Alleviation of the Common Cold
Improving Sleep depth and length
Detoxing and Cleasning the body
Improving Bones Teeth Nerves and Muscle

Buckwheat and **Quinoa**: Too high in carbs to be included in our list and not suitable for a Blender Recipe

Chili Peppers and Garlic: Great but not really suitable for a Blender Recipe

Almonds: High in Protein, unsaturated Fat, Vitamins B1, B2, B3, B9, E, Calcium, Copper, Iron, Magnesium Phosphorus, Potassium, Zinc and Fibre

Dark Cholcolate: High in Protein, Saturated Fat, Vitamins B1, B2, B3, B9, K, Calcium, Copper, Magnesium Manganese, Phosphorus, Potassium, Selenium, Zinc and Fibre

Flax Seeds: High in Protein, unsaturated Fat, Vitamins B1, B3, B5, B6, B9, Calcium, Copper, Iron, Magnesium, Manganese, Phosphorus, Potassium, Selenium, Zinc, Fibre

Pumpkin Seeds: High in Protein,unsaturated Fat, Vitamins B2, B3, B5, B6, B9, E, Calcium, Copper, Iron, Magnesium, Manganese, Phosphorus, Potassium, Selenium, Zinc

Chia Seeds: High in Protein, has all essential amino acids in good quantity, incredibly high in Fibre at 34%, High in Omega3 at 17%, Vitamins B1, B2, B3, B9, Calcium, Copper Manganese, Phosphorus, Selenium, Zinc

Apricots: High in Vitamins A.C, E, Iron, Potassium, Fibre

Avocados: High in unsaturated Fat, Vitamins B2, B3, B5, B6, B9, C, K Cooper, Magnesium, Manganese and Potassium, Fibre

Blueberries: High in Vitamins B9, C, K, Manganese and Fibre

Raspberries: High in Vitamins B1, B2, B3, B9, C, K, Copper, Iron, Manganese and Fibre

Blackberries: High in Vitamins B9, C, K, Manganese and Fibre

Guavas: High in Vitamins: A, B9, C, Copper, Magnesium, Manganese, Potassium, Fibre

Papaya: High in Vitamins A, B9, C, Potassium, Fiber

Goji Berries: Contains all 11 Essential amino Acids - High in Vitamins A B2 C, Calcium, Selenium, Zinc, Iron, Potassium. But 46% Sugars. So not too many of them. Cures everything from impotence to malaria according to internet hype. Waitrose do them in the UK. Also called Wolfberries

Ginger: High in Vitamins B1, B2, B5, B6, C, Calcium, Copper, Iron, Magnesium, Manganese, Potassium, Selenium, Zinc, Fibre

Broccoli: High in Vitamins A, B1, B2, B5, B6, B9, C, K, Calcium, Iron, Magnesium, Manganese, Potassium

Carrots: High in Vitamins A, B3, B6, B9, C, K, Manganese, Potassium, Fibre

Tomatoes: High in Vitamins A, B2, B6, B9 C, Potassium, Lycopene

Beetroot: Vitamin B6, B9, C, Iron, Magnesium, Manganese, Phosphorus, Potassium, Zinc, Fibre

Kale: High in Vitamins A, B1, B2, B3, B6, B9, C, K, Calcium, Copper, Iron, Magnesium, Manganese, Potassium

Spinach: High in Vitamins A, B2, B6, B9, C, E, K, Calcium, Copper, Iron. Magnesium, Manganese, Potassium, Fibre

Swiss Chard: High in Vitamins A, C, E, K, Calcium, Copper, Iron, Magensium, Manganese, Potassium, Sodium

Hence we include many Superfood Blast and Smoothie Recipes!

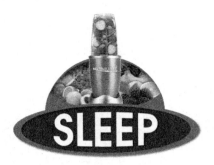

Sleep and Foods

As an example of what food can do for you - here is how diet can help you sleep - without having to take sleeping tablets. If you suffer from insomnia then you may be deficient in an essential amino acid called Tryptophan.

The key players in putting your body to sleep are Serotonin, Melatonin and Tryptophan. All of these can be purchased from health food shops.

The chemical pathway works like this. First the body converts Tryptophan into Tryptophan Hydroxylase (or 5 HydroxyTryptophan or 5HTP). Then this, together with Vitamins. B3, B6, B9 and Magnesium is used to synthesize the neurotransmitter Serotonin. The Serotonin is then converted to the neurohormone Melatonin as necessary

Serotonin is the body's natural sedative. The higher your serotonin levels are the more sleepy you feel. Melatonin controls your body clock, your circadian rhythm, your sleep cycle. These two hormones both put you to sleep and determine how long and how good your sleep quality is.

Tryptophan is one of the essential amino acids – which means that it is essential for human life and the body cannot manufacture it. So we have to eat it!

Just taking 1 gram of Tryptophan can significantly decrease the time it takes to fall asleep and the time you stay asleep for. 6 grams are used to treat certain forms of PMS. 3 grams per day for 2 weeks is prescribed to treat depression and anxiety without the side effects associated with clinical anti depressants like Prosac.So to cheer yourself up eat some foods which are rich in Tryptophan!

Foods which are high in Tryptophan include Chocolate, Eggs, Cheese, Brown rice, Avocados, Walnuts, Peanuts, Meats, Sesame seeds, Sunflower seeds and Pumpkin seeds. So having a cup of cocoa before you go to bed has a sound basis in biochemistry!

Best Seeds	Tryptophan /100g	Best Greens	Tryptophan /100g
Chia Seeds	721 mg	Parsely	45 mg
Pumpkin Seeds	576 mg	Spinach	39 mg
Sesame Seeds	388 mg	Kale	34 mg
Sunflower Seeds	348 mg	Broccoli	33 mg
Flax Seed	297 mg	Watercress	30 mg
		Swiss Chard	17 mg
		Bok Choy	15 mg

Best Nuts	Tryptophan /100g	Best Veggies	Tryptophan /100g
Cashew Nuts	470 mg	Cauliflower	20 mg
Peanuts	340 mg	Beetroot	19 mg
Walnuts	318 mg	Fine Beans	19 mg
Pistachio Nuts	284 mg	Carrot	12 mg
Almonds	214 mg	Zucchini	10 mg
Hazelnuts	193 mg		
Brazil Nuts	141 mg		
Pecans	93 mg		

Best Fruits	Tryptophan /100g	Foods	Tryptophan /100g
Avocado	26 mg	Cocoa Powder	283 mg
Prunes	25 mg	Dairy Milk	40 mg
Apricots	12 mg	Cheddar Cheese	515 mg
Dates	12 mg	Mozarella Cheese	558 mg
Grapes	11 mg	Egg	210 mg
Oranges	10 mg		
Peaches	10 mg		
Plums	9 mg		
Grapefruits	9 mg		

Some of our NutriBullet Recipes are designed to deliver Tryptophan. The RDI is 285 mg. But for a good nights sleep 1000 mg is better. Lots of Chia seeds Cashews Milk Spinach and Prunes and some Cocoa powder will get you to around 475 mg of Tryptophan from one NutriBlast. That is 166% of the RDI. But you would need 2 of them to really help with sleep that night. Alternatively eat 100 gram of cheese, that would give you another 500 mg of Tryptophan.

Game meat poultry and eggs are also great non nutribullet sources of Tryptophan. If you need something stronger then consider taking the intermediary between Tryptophan and Serotonin - 5HTP as a supplement. Double-blind studies have shown that 5HTP is as effective as Prozac, Paxil, Zoloft, Imipramine and Desipramine and it has less side effects being a natural body compound. 5HTP is cheaper and non prescription being a regular dietary supplement.

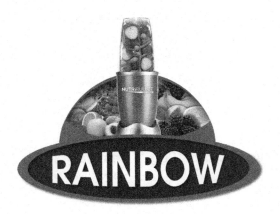

Eat a Rainbow of Colour

Red – Lyopene, anthocyanins and other phytonutrients found in red fruits and veggies. Lycopene is a powerful antioxidant that can help reduce the risk of cancer and keep our heart healthy and improve memory function.

White/Tan – Contrary to popular belief, white foods aren't so useless after all! These foods have been shown to reduce the risk of certain cancers, balance hormone levels, lower blood pressure, and boost your body's natural immunity with nutrients such as EGCG and allicin. White fruits and vegetables contain a range of health-promoting phytochemicals such as allicin (found in garlic) which is known for its antiviral and antibacterial properties. Some members of the white group, such as bananas and potatoes, are also a good source of potassium.

Green – Chlorophyll-rich detoxification properties are the most noted value in leafy greens. In addition, luteins, zeaxanthin, along with indoles, help boost greens' cancer-fighting properties, encourage vision health, and help build strong bones and teeth. Green vegetables contain a range of phytochemicals including carotenoids, indoles and saponins, all of which have anti-cancer properties. Leafy greens such as spinach and broccoli are also excellent sources of folate.

Blue/Purple – Phytochemicals anthocyanin and resveratrol promote youthful skin, hair and nails. In addition, these anti-inflammatory compounds may also play a role in cancer-prevention, especially skin cancer and urinary and digestive tract health. They may also reduce the risk of cardio vascular disease.

Orange/Yellow – Foods glowing with orange and yellow are great immune-boosters and vision protectors, mainly due to their high levels of carotenoids. Carotenoids give this group their vibrant colour. A well-known carotenoid called Betacarotene is found in sweet potatoes, pumpkins and carrots. It is converted to vitamin A, which helps maintain healthy mucous membranes and healthy eyes. Another carotenoid called lutein is stored in the eye and has been found to prevent cataracts and age-related macular degeneration, which can lead to blindness.

Eat Organic?

Organic fruits and vegetables generally have around 33% of the man-made pesticide residues found on non-organic varieties. Some studies have shown that they have more anti-oxidants but less protein than their chemically treated cousins. But the differences are too small to have a significant impact on nutrition. However the organically grown varieties are attacked by the very same pests as their non organic relatives and so do not sit idly by taking that attack without responding chemically. They either produce natural pesticides which could be toxic to humans or they can be damaged from the attack and that damage can produce toxins. Also organic food without preservatives will become damaged by micro-organisms more quickly than food with preservatives. It then becomes a question of whether that microbial damage is a larger health risk than the preservative is! So the best thing to do is to wash all fruits and vegetables – whether organic or non organic in order to remove whatever residues they have.

Scientifically there is not yet enough evidence on the long term effect upon human health to say statistically that organic food is better for you. Furthermore the most contaminated places in a building are the door handles and elevator buttons because these are touched by the largest number of people. So if fruit is on display in a supermarket, the largest contaminant might be those who have touched that fruit and squeezed it before you purchase it. It therefore follows that online purchasing might be healthier than supermarket display purchasing. So perhaps it is better to make you own decision based upon the quality of the food you see in front of you rather than relying upon an organic label procured from a government department?

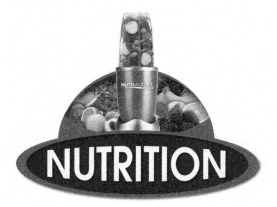

Nutrition Data

All our Blasts and Smoothies come with full nutritional data giving the precise number of grams of Protein, Carbohydrate, Fat and Fibre for each recipe and the number of Kcals it contains. The data is taken mainly from the USDA database.

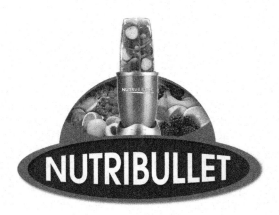

NutriBullet Capacities

US traditional cup is 8 US fluid oz or 240 ml (236 ml to be exact). However putting berries or slices or cubes of fruit and veggies into a cup wastes around 50% of the space so in weight terms an 8 fluid oz cup will contain around 4 oz or 120 grams of contents.

Greens use even less of the space, so 1 Cups/Handfuls of Spinach or Kale will only weigh around 40 grams or 1½ oz – even after pressing it down a bit.

There are 28.35 grams in a British Imperial fluid ounce, which is 4% larger than the US fluid ounce - which is pretty unhelpful. So it is easier just to take 28 grams for an ounce in both cases.

The NutriBullet tall cup takes 590 ml/grams of water up to the MAX fill line. The small cup takes 305 grams of water up to the MAX fill line.

All our recipes are designed and stated for the standard tall cup (28 oz total, 24 oz to max fill). *To use the small cup you just halve them all!*

The entire tall cup can take around 826 ml/grams of water up to the top. This is 3½ standard US cups or 28 fluid ounces. However we can put 4¼ cups worth of greens, veggies, fruits, nuts and seeds into the tall cup because they compress a lot when they lose their shape after blasting. All ingredients are stated in Cups and Handfuls or Grams and American Ounces (oz)

Warnings

Do not put your hand or any implement near the blades when the NutriBullet is plugged in to an electricity supply.

Cleaning

The NutriBullet is easy to clean. The manufacturers recommend warm water (not hot) and a mild detergent. Rinse the blades and the cups and the base (if necessary) immediately after use to prevent the debris from drying.

Authors Preference for Kale

Kale is a Superfood and is very good for you. But it does not taste as good as the other greens in a NutriBlast in our opinion! To be frank, it tastes like cardboard. So we have excluded it from these recipes. It is better to fry it in some olive oil or roast it in the oven and make lovely Kale chips. If you can stand the taste of it then feel free to swap one of the greens in any recipe for Kale!

AVOID THESE INGREDIENTS: Apple Pear Peach Plum Apricot and Cherry **stones and pips** contain cyanide which is very poisonous. These stones and pips *must* therefore be removed before use!

Rhubarb leaves contain oxalate which causes kidney stones, comas, convulsions. 5lb of Rhubarb leaves is fatal!

Tomatoes are fine but the **tomato leaves and vines** are not. They contain alkaloid poisons such as atropine which causes headaches dizziness and vomiting.

Nutmeg: Contains myristicine which is halucingoenic and causes dizziness and vomiting. It is OK in small quantities as a spice but we do not recommend it for the NutriBullet.

Kidney Beans and **Lima Beans**: These are really really poisonous if eaten raw.

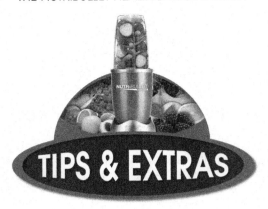

Tips and Extras

Cinnamon and Cloves are lovely in a hot drink but do not really work in a cold one such as a Nutribullet blast. We cannot recommend adding sugar given the health difficulties associated with refined sucrose. But the following are fantastic in Nutriblasts…

Ginger Root (sliced)
Lemon Juice
Lime Juice
Agave Nectar
Honey
Garlic Cloves
Cocoa Powder which is also called Cacao Powder (a Superfood)
85% Dark Chocolate (a Superfood)
Maca Powder (a Superfood)
Instant Coffee
Coriander
Parsley
Sage
Chives
Chlorella Powder (Detoxing supergreen 50% protein algae)
Spirulina Powder (Supergreen immunity boosting 57% protein algae)
Whey Protein Powder (Banana, Chocolate, Cookies, Strawberry flavours etc.) – for extra protein
Rice Protein Powder
Pea Protein Powder
Soy Protein Powder

These can be added to any of the recipes for a taste or nutrition boost.

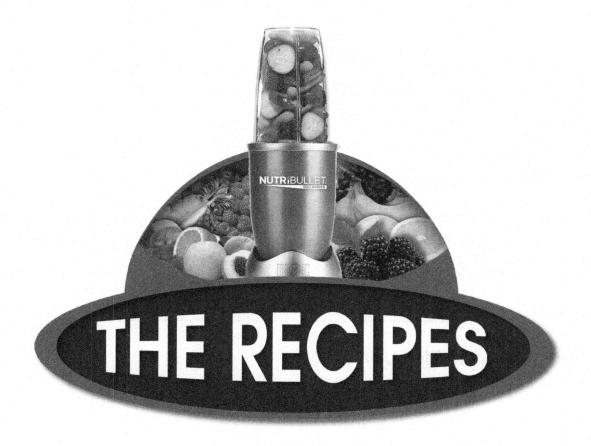

Spinach Royale

Ingredients

1 Cup/Handful of Spinach (40 grams or 1½ oz)
1 Cup/Handful of Swiss Chard (40 grams or 1½ oz)
1 Cup of Guava (120 grams or 4 oz)
½ Cup of Goji Berries Dried (40 grams or 1½ oz)
22 grams or ¾ oz of Chia Seeds
200 ml / 7 fl oz of Almond Milk (Unsweetened)

Protein 15g, Fat 11g, Carb 37g, Fibre 18g, 359 Kcals

Preparation

Place the nuts or seeds into the Tall Cup. Screw the Nutribullet Extractor Blade on to the top of the cup. Invert the cup, press it down into the Nutribullet Power Base and twist it into place. Blast them for 30 seconds. Put the rest of the solid ingredients into the cup and press them down below the Max Line. Add the fluid base to fill the cup up to the Max Line. Screw the Nutribullet Extractor Blade on to the top of the cup. Invert the cup, press it down into the Nutribullet Power Base and twist it into place. Blast the mixture until it is really smooth (20 or so seconds). **Enjoy!**

Papaya goes Blueberry

Ingredients

2 Cups/Handfuls of Broccoli Florets (80 grams or 3 oz)
1 Cup of Papaya (120 grams or 4 oz)
1 Cup of Blueberries (120 grams or 4 oz)
30 grams or 1 oz of Almonds
200 ml / 7 fl oz of Water

Protein 10g, Fat 17g, Carb 31g, Fibre 10g, 324 Kcals

Preparation

Place the nuts or seeds into the Tall Cup. Screw the Nutribullet Extractor Blade on to the top of the cup. Invert the cup, press it down into the Nutribullet Power Base and twist it into place. Blast them for 30 seconds. Put the rest of the solid ingredients into the cup and press them down below the Max Line. Add the fluid base to fill the cup up to the Max Line. Screw the Nutribullet Extractor Blade on to the top of the cup. Invert the cup, press it down into the Nutribullet Power Base and twist it into place. Blast the mixture until it is really smooth (20 or so seconds). **Enjoy!**

Broccoli in Avocado

Ingredients

1 Cup/Handful of Broccoli Florets (40 grams or 1½ oz)
1 Cup/Handful of Spinach (40 grams or 1½ oz)
1 small Avocado (stoned and peeled) (120 grams or 4 oz)
1 Cup of Apricot halves (120 grams or 4 oz)
22 grams or ¾ oz of Flax Seeds
200 ml / 7 fl oz of Dairy Milk Whole

Protein 17g, Fat 35g, Carb 25g, Fibre 18g, 517 Kcals

Preparation

Place the nuts or seeds into the Tall Cup. Screw the Nutribullet Extractor Blade on to the top of the cup. Invert the cup, press it down into the Nutribullet Power Base and twist it into place. Blast them for 30 seconds. Put the rest of the solid ingredients into the cup and press them down below the Max Line. Add the fluid base to fill the cup up to the Max Line. Screw the Nutribullet Extractor Blade on to the top of the cup. Invert the cup, press it down into the Nutribullet Power Base and twist it into place. Blast the mixture until it is really smooth (20 or so seconds). ***Enjoy!***

Broccoli kisses Chard

Ingredients

1 Cup/Handful of Broccoli Florets (40 grams or 1½ oz)
1 Cup/Handful of Swiss Chard (40 grams or 1½ oz)
1 Cup of Blackberries (120 grams or 4 oz)
1 Cup of Raspberries (120 grams or 4 oz)
22 grams or ¾ oz of Pumpkin Seeds
200 ml / 7 fl oz of Dairy Milk Whole

Protein 17g, Fat 18g, Carb 26g, Fibre 17g, 387 Kcals

Preparation

Place the nuts or seeds into the Tall Cup. Screw the Nutribullet Extractor Blade on to the top of the cup. Invert the cup, press it down into the Nutribullet Power Base and twist it into place. Blast them for 30 seconds. Put the rest of the solid ingredients into the cup and press them down below the Max Line. Add the fluid base to fill the cup up to the Max Line. Screw the Nutribullet Extractor Blade on to the top of the cup. Invert the cup, press it down into the Nutribullet Power Base and twist it into place. Blast the mixture until it is really smooth (20 or so seconds). ***Enjoy!***

Chard invites Goji

Ingredients

1 Cup/Handful of Swiss Chard (40 grams or 1½ oz)
1 Cup/Handful of Spinach (40 grams or 1½ oz)
½ Cup of Goji Berries Dried (40 grams or 1½ oz)
1 small Avocado (stoned and peeled) (120 grams or 4 oz)
22 grams or ¾ oz of Chia Seeds
200 ml / 7 fl oz of Almond Milk (Unsweetened)

Protein 14g, Fat 28g, Carb 28g, Fibre 20g, 470 Kcals

Preparation

Place the nuts or seeds into the Tall Cup. Screw the Nutribullet Extractor Blade on to the top of the cup. Invert the cup, press it down into the Nutribullet Power Base and twist it into place. Blast them for 30 seconds. Put the rest of the solid ingredients into the cup and press them down below the Max Line. Add the fluid base to fill the cup up to the Max Line. Screw the Nutribullet Extractor Blade on to the top of the cup. Invert the cup, press it down into the Nutribullet Power Base and twist it into place. Blast the mixture until it is really smooth (20 or so seconds). **Enjoy!**

Papaya and Flax Salad

Ingredients

1 Cup/Handful of Broccoli Florets (40 grams or 1½ oz)
1 Cup/Handful of Swiss Chard (40 grams or 1½ oz)
2 Cups of Papaya (240 grams or 8 oz)
22 grams or ¾ oz of Flax Seeds
200 ml / 7 fl oz of Water

Protein 7g, Fat 10g, Carb 25g, Fibre 12g, 241 Kcals

Preparation

Place the nuts or seeds into the Tall Cup. Screw the Nutribullet Extractor Blade on to the top of the cup. Invert the cup, press it down into the Nutribullet Power Base and twist it into place. Blast them for 30 seconds. Put the rest of the solid ingredients into the cup and press them down below the Max Line. Add the fluid base to fill the cup up to the Max Line. Screw the Nutribullet Extractor Blade on to the top of the cup. Invert the cup, press it down into the Nutribullet Power Base and twist it into place. Blast the mixture until it is really smooth (20 or so seconds). **Enjoy!**

Broccoli befriends Pumpkin

Ingredients

1 Cup/Handful of Broccoli Florets (40 grams or 1½ oz)
1 Cup/Handful of Spinach (40 grams or 1½ oz)
1 Cup of Blackberries (120 grams or 4 oz)
1 Cup of Apricot halves (120 grams or 4 oz)
22 grams or ¾ oz of Pumpkin Seeds
200 ml / 7 fl oz of Almond Milk (Unsweetened)

Protein 12g, Fat 13g, Carb 21g, Fibre 13g, 282 Kcals

Preparation

Place the nuts or seeds into the Tall Cup. Screw the Nutribullet Extractor Blade on to the top of the cup. Invert the cup, press it down into the Nutribullet Power Base and twist it into place. Blast them for 30 seconds. Put the rest of the solid ingredients into the cup and press them down below the Max Line. Add the fluid base to fill the cup up to the Max Line. Screw the Nutribullet Extractor Blade on to the top of the cup. Invert the cup, press it down into the Nutribullet Power Base and twist it into place. Blast the mixture until it is really smooth (20 or so seconds). *Enjoy!*

Chard Paradise

Ingredients

1 Cup/Handful of Spinach (40 grams or 1½ oz)
1 Cup/Handful of Swiss Chard (40 grams or 1½ oz)
1 Cup of Raspberries (120 grams or 4 oz)
1 Cup of Papaya (120 grams or 4 oz)
30 grams or 1 oz of Almonds
200 ml / 7 fl oz of Water

Protein 10g, Fat 17g, Carb 21g, Fibre 14g, 307 Kcals

Preparation

Place the nuts or seeds into the Tall Cup. Screw the Nutribullet Extractor Blade on to the top of the cup. Invert the cup, press it down into the Nutribullet Power Base and twist it into place. Blast them for 30 seconds. Put the rest of the solid ingredients into the cup and press them down below the Max Line. Add the fluid base to fill the cup up to the Max Line. Screw the Nutribullet Extractor Blade on to the top of the cup. Invert the cup, press it down into the Nutribullet Power Base and twist it into place. Blast the mixture until it is really smooth (20 or so seconds). *Enjoy!*

Broccoli partners Blueberry

Ingredients

1 Cup/Handful of Broccoli Florets (40 grams or 1½ oz)
1 Cup/Handful of Spinach (40 grams or 1½ oz)
1 Cup of Blueberries (120 grams or 4 oz)
1 Cup of Guava (120 grams or 4 oz)
22 grams or ¾ oz of Chia Seeds
200 ml / 7 fl oz of Dairy Milk Whole

Protein 16g, Fat 16g, Carb 38g, Fibre 19g, 407 Kcals

Preparation

Place the nuts or seeds into the Tall Cup. Screw the Nutribullet Extractor Blade on to the top of the cup. Invert the cup, press it down into the Nutribullet Power Base and twist it into place. Blast them for 30 seconds. Put the rest of the solid ingredients into the cup and press them down below the Max Line. Add the fluid base to fill the cup up to the Max Line. Screw the Nutribullet Extractor Blade on to the top of the cup. Invert the cup, press it down into the Nutribullet Power Base and twist it into place. Blast the mixture until it is really smooth (20 or so seconds). ***Enjoy!***

Blueberry joins Flax

Ingredients

1 Cup/Handful of Swiss Chard (40 grams or 1½ oz)
1 Cup/Handful of Broccoli Florets (40 grams or 1½ oz)
2 Cups of Blueberries (240 grams or 8 oz)
22 grams or ¾ oz of Flax Seeds
200 ml / 7 fl oz of Dairy Milk Whole

Protein 14g, Fat 18g, Carb 41g, Fibre 13g, 403 Kcals

Preparation

Place the nuts or seeds into the Tall Cup. Screw the Nutribullet Extractor Blade on to the top of the cup. Invert the cup, press it down into the Nutribullet Power Base and twist it into place. Blast them for 30 seconds. Put the rest of the solid ingredients into the cup and press them down below the Max Line. Add the fluid base to fill the cup up to the Max Line. Screw the Nutribullet Extractor Blade on to the top of the cup. Invert the cup, press it down into the Nutribullet Power Base and twist it into place. Blast the mixture until it is really smooth (20 or so seconds). ***Enjoy!***

Chia Orchard

Ingredients

2 Cups/Handfuls of Broccoli Florets (80 grams or 3 oz)
1 Cup of Papaya (120 grams or 4 oz)
1 Cup of diced Beetroot (120 grams or 4 oz)
22 grams or ¾ oz of Chia Seeds
200 ml / 7 fl oz of Water

Protein 8g, Fat 8g, Carb 24g, Fibre 15g, 237 Kcals

Preparation

Place the nuts or seeds into the Tall Cup. Screw the Nutribullet Extractor Blade on to the top of the cup. Invert the cup, press it down into the Nutribullet Power Base and twist it into place. Blast them for 30 seconds. Put the rest of the solid ingredients into the cup and press them down below the Max Line. Add the fluid base to fill the cup up to the Max Line. Screw the Nutribullet Extractor Blade on to the top of the cup. Invert the cup, press it down into the Nutribullet Power Base and twist it into place. Blast the mixture until it is really smooth (20 or so seconds). **Enjoy!**

Guava Blend

Ingredients

1 Cup/Handful of Spinach (40 grams or 1½ oz)
1 Cup/Handful of Broccoli Florets (40 grams or 1½ oz)
1 Cup of Guava (120 grams or 4 oz)
1 Cup of sliced Carrots (120 grams or 4 oz)
22 grams or ¾ oz of Pumpkin Seeds
200 ml / 7 fl oz of Dairy Milk Whole

Protein 18g, Fat 19g, Carb 33g, Fibre 13g, 405 Kcals

Preparation

Place the nuts or seeds into the Tall Cup. Screw the Nutribullet Extractor Blade on to the top of the cup. Invert the cup, press it down into the Nutribullet Power Base and twist it into place. Blast them for 30 seconds. Put the rest of the solid ingredients into the cup and press them down below the Max Line. Add the fluid base to fill the cup up to the Max Line. Screw the Nutribullet Extractor Blade on to the top of the cup. Invert the cup, press it down into the Nutribullet Power Base and twist it into place. Blast the mixture until it is really smooth (20 or so seconds). **Enjoy!**

Tomato Soother

Ingredients

1 Cup/Handful of Swiss Chard (40 grams or 1½ oz)
1 Cup/Handful of Spinach (40 grams or 1½ oz)
1 Cup of Raspberries (120 grams or 4 oz)
1 Cup of sliced Tomato (120 grams or 4 oz)
30 grams or 1 oz of Almonds
200 ml / 7 fl oz of Almond Milk (Unsweetened)

Protein 12g, Fat 19g, Carb 13g, Fibre 15g, 303 Kcals

Preparation

Place the nuts or seeds into the Tall Cup. Screw the Nutribullet Extractor Blade on to the top of the cup. Invert the cup, press it down into the Nutribullet Power Base and twist it into place. Blast them for 30 seconds. Put the rest of the solid ingredients into the cup and press them down below the Max Line. Add the fluid base to fill the cup up to the Max Line. Screw the Nutribullet Extractor Blade on to the top of the cup. Invert the cup, press it down into the Nutribullet Power Base and twist it into place. Blast the mixture until it is really smooth (20 or so seconds). **Enjoy!**

Broccoli Sunshine

Ingredients

1 Cup/Handful of Broccoli Florets (40 grams or 1½ oz)
1 Cup/Handful of Swiss Chard (40 grams or 1½ oz)
1 Cup of Blackberries (120 grams or 4 oz)
1 Cup of sliced Tomato (120 grams or 4 oz)
22 grams or ¾ oz of Flax Seeds
200 ml / 7 fl oz of Water

Protein 9g, Fat 10g, Carb 11g, Fibre 15g, 211 Kcals

Preparation

Place the nuts or seeds into the Tall Cup. Screw the Nutribullet Extractor Blade on to the top of the cup. Invert the cup, press it down into the Nutribullet Power Base and twist it into place. Blast them for 30 seconds. Put the rest of the solid ingredients into the cup and press them down below the Max Line. Add the fluid base to fill the cup up to the Max Line. Screw the Nutribullet Extractor Blade on to the top of the cup. Invert the cup, press it down into the Nutribullet Power Base and twist it into place. Blast the mixture until it is really smooth (20 or so seconds). **Enjoy!**

Flax Supermodel

Ingredients

1 Cup/Handful of Swiss Chard (40 grams or 1½ oz)
1 Cup/Handful of Spinach (40 grams or 1½ oz)
1 small Avocado (stoned and peeled) (120 grams or 4 oz)
1 Cup of diced Beetroot (120 grams or 4 oz)
22 grams or ¾ oz of Flax Seeds
200 ml / 7 fl oz of Almond Milk (Unsweetened)

Protein 11g, Fat 30g, Carb 12g, Fibre 20g, 403 Kcals

Preparation

Place the nuts or seeds into the Tall Cup. Screw the Nutribullet Extractor Blade on to the top of the cup. Invert the cup, press it down into the Nutribullet Power Base and twist it into place. Blast them for 30 seconds. Put the rest of the solid ingredients into the cup and press them down below the Max Line. Add the fluid base to fill the cup up to the Max Line. Screw the Nutribullet Extractor Blade on to the top of the cup. Invert the cup, press it down into the Nutribullet Power Base and twist it into place. Blast the mixture until it is really smooth (20 or so seconds). *Enjoy!*

Blueberry Explosion

Ingredients

2 Cups/Handfuls of Spinach (80 grams or 3 oz)
1 Cup of Blueberries (120 grams or 4 oz)
1 Cup of sliced Carrots (120 grams or 4 oz)
22 grams or ¾ oz of Pumpkin Seeds
200 ml / 7 fl oz of Dairy Milk Whole

Protein 16g, Fat 18g, Carb 35g, Fibre 9g, 388 Kcals

Preparation

Place the nuts or seeds into the Tall Cup. Screw the Nutribullet Extractor Blade on to the top of the cup. Invert the cup, press it down into the Nutribullet Power Base and twist it into place. Blast them for 30 seconds. Put the rest of the solid ingredients into the cup and press them down below the Max Line. Add the fluid base to fill the cup up to the Max Line. Screw the Nutribullet Extractor Blade on to the top of the cup. Invert the cup, press it down into the Nutribullet Power Base and twist it into place. Blast the mixture until it is really smooth (20 or so seconds). *Enjoy!*

Broccoli hugs Apricot

Ingredients

2 Cups/Handfuls of Broccoli Florets (80 grams or 3 oz)
1 Cup of Apricot halves (120 grams or 4 oz)
1 Cup of sliced Tomato (120 grams or 4 oz)
22 grams or ¾ oz of Chia Seeds
200 ml / 7 fl oz of Dairy Milk Whole

Protein 15g, Fat 15g, Carb 29g, Fibre 13g, 341 Kcals

Preparation

Place the nuts or seeds into the Tall Cup. Screw the Nutribullet Extractor Blade on to the top of the cup. Invert the cup, press it down into the Nutribullet Power Base and twist it into place. Blast them for 30 seconds. Put the rest of the solid ingredients into the cup and press them down below the Max Line. Add the fluid base to fill the cup up to the Max Line. Screw the Nutribullet Extractor Blade on to the top of the cup. Invert the cup, press it down into the Nutribullet Power Base and twist it into place. Blast the mixture until it is really smooth (20 or so seconds). **Enjoy!**

Beetroot Delivered

Ingredients

1 Cup/Handful of Broccoli Florets (40 grams or 1½ oz)
1 Cup/Handful of Swiss Chard (40 grams or 1½ oz)
½ Cup of Goji Berries Dried (40 grams or 1½ oz)
1 Cup of diced Beetroot (120 grams or 4 oz)
30 grams or 1 oz of Almonds
200 ml / 7 fl oz of Almond Milk (Unsweetened)

Protein 17g, Fat 19g, Carb 36g, Fibre 11g, 404 Kcals

Preparation

Place the nuts or seeds into the Tall Cup. Screw the Nutribullet Extractor Blade on to the top of the cup. Invert the cup, press it down into the Nutribullet Power Base and twist it into place. Blast them for 30 seconds. Put the rest of the solid ingredients into the cup and press them down below the Max Line. Add the fluid base to fill the cup up to the Max Line. Screw the Nutribullet Extractor Blade on to the top of the cup. Invert the cup, press it down into the Nutribullet Power Base and twist it into place. Blast the mixture until it is really smooth (20 or so seconds). **Enjoy!**

Chard Twist

Ingredients

2 Cups/Handfuls of Swiss Chard (80 grams or 3 oz)
1 Cup of Guava (120 grams or 4 oz)
1 Cup of sliced Carrots (120 grams or 4 oz)
30 grams or 1 oz of Almonds
200 ml / 7 fl oz of Water

Protein 12g, Fat 17g, Carb 23g, Fibre 14g, 322 Kcals

Preparation

Place the nuts or seeds into the Tall Cup. Screw the Nutribullet Extractor Blade on to the top of the cup. Invert the cup, press it down into the Nutribullet Power Base and twist it into place. Blast them for 30 seconds. Put the rest of the solid ingredients into the cup and press them down below the Max Line. Add the fluid base to fill the cup up to the Max Line. Screw the Nutribullet Extractor Blade on to the top of the cup. Invert the cup, press it down into the Nutribullet Power Base and twist it into place. Blast the mixture until it is really smooth (20 or so seconds). ***Enjoy!***

Goji kisses Flax

Ingredients

2 Cups/Handfuls of Swiss Chard (80 grams or 3 oz)
½ Cup of Goji Berries Dried (40 grams or 1½ oz)
1 Cup of sliced Tomato (120 grams or 4 oz)
22 grams or ¾ oz of Flax Seeds
200 ml / 7 fl oz of Water

Protein 12g, Fat 10g, Carb 28g, Fibre 11g, 282 Kcals

Preparation

Place the nuts or seeds into the Tall Cup. Screw the Nutribullet Extractor Blade on to the top of the cup. Invert the cup, press it down into the Nutribullet Power Base and twist it into place. Blast them for 30 seconds. Put the rest of the solid ingredients into the cup and press them down below the Max Line. Add the fluid base to fill the cup up to the Max Line. Screw the Nutribullet Extractor Blade on to the top of the cup. Invert the cup, press it down into the Nutribullet Power Base and twist it into place. Blast the mixture until it is really smooth (20 or so seconds). ***Enjoy!***

Blackberry and Goji Potion

Ingredients

1 Cup/Handful of Spinach (40 grams or 1½ oz)
1 Cup/Handful of Swiss Chard (40 grams or 1½ oz)
1 Cup of Blackberries (120 grams or 4 oz)
½ Cup of Goji Berries Dried (40 grams or 1½ oz)
200 ml / 7 fl oz of Dairy Milk Whole

Protein 16g, Fat 9g, Carb 39g, Fibre 10g, 324 Kcals

Preparation

Put all the solid ingredients into the Tall Cup and press them down below the Max Line. Add the fluid base to fill the cup up to the Max Line. Screw the Nutribullet Extractor Blade on to the top of the cup. Invert the cup, press it down into the Nutribullet Power Base and twist it into place. Blast the mixture until it is really smooth (20 or so seconds). *Enjoy!*

Broccoli in Spinach

Ingredients

1 Cup/Handful of Broccoli Florets (40 grams or 1½ oz)
1 Cup/Handful of Spinach (40 grams or 1½ oz)
1 Cup of Raspberries (120 grams or 4 oz)
1 Cup of Apricot halves (120 grams or 4 oz)
200 ml / 7 fl oz of Water

Protein 5g, Fat 2g, Carb 20g, Fibre 12g, 142 Kcals

Preparation

Put all the solid ingredients into the Tall Cup and press them down below the Max Line. Add the fluid base to fill the cup up to the Max Line. Screw the Nutribullet Extractor Blade on to the top of the cup. Invert the cup, press it down into the Nutribullet Power Base and twist it into place. Blast the mixture until it is really smooth (20 or so seconds). *Enjoy!*

Papaya Delivered

Ingredients

2 Cups/Handfuls of Spinach (80 grams or 3 oz)
1 Cup of Papaya (120 grams or 4 oz)
1 Cup of Guava (120 grams or 4 oz)
200 ml / 7 fl oz of Almond Milk (Unsweetened)

Protein 7g, Fat 4g, Carb 23g, Fibre 11g, 177 Kcals

Preparation

Put all the solid ingredients into the Tall Cup and press them down below the Max Line. Add the fluid base to fill the cup up to the Max Line. Screw the Nutribullet Extractor Blade on to the top of the cup. Invert the cup, press it down into the Nutribullet Power Base and twist it into place. Blast the mixture until it is really smooth (20 or so seconds). *Enjoy!*

Avocado Seduction

Ingredients

1 Cup/Handful of Swiss Chard (40 grams or 1½ oz)
1 Cup/Handful of Broccoli Florets (40 grams or 1½ oz)
1 Cup of Blueberries (120 grams or 4 oz)
1 small Avocado (stoned and peeled) (120 grams or 4 oz)
200 ml / 7 fl oz of Dairy Milk Whole

Protein 12g, Fat 25g, Carb 29g, Fibre 13g, 409 Kcals

Preparation

Put all the solid ingredients into the Tall Cup and press them down below the Max Line. Add the fluid base to fill the cup up to the Max Line. Screw the Nutribullet Extractor Blade on to the top of the cup. Invert the cup, press it down into the Nutribullet Power Base and twist it into place. Blast the mixture until it is really smooth (20 or so seconds). *Enjoy!*

Broccoli Concerto

Ingredients

1 Cup/Handful of Broccoli Florets (40 grams or 1½ oz)
1 Cup/Handful of Swiss Chard (40 grams or 1½ oz)
1 small Avocado (stoned and peeled) (120 grams or 4 oz)
1 Cup of Apricot halves (120 grams or 4 oz)
200 ml / 7 fl oz of Water

Protein 6g, Fat 18g, Carb 16g, Fibre 12g, 270 Kcals

Preparation

Put all the solid ingredients into the Tall Cup and press them down below the Max Line. Add the fluid base to fill the cup up to the Max Line. Screw the Nutribullet Extractor Blade on to the top of the cup. Invert the cup, press it down into the Nutribullet Power Base and twist it into place. Blast the mixture until it is really smooth (20 or so seconds). **Enjoy!**

Papaya hugs Guava

Ingredients

1 Cup/Handful of Spinach (40 grams or 1½ oz)
1 Cup/Handful of Swiss Chard (40 grams or 1½ oz)
1 Cup of Papaya (120 grams or 4 oz)
1 Cup of Guava (120 grams or 4 oz)
200 ml / 7 fl oz of Almond Milk (Unsweetened)

Protein 6g, Fat 4g, Carb 23g, Fibre 11g, 175 Kcals

Preparation

Put all the solid ingredients into the Tall Cup and press them down below the Max Line. Add the fluid base to fill the cup up to the Max Line. Screw the Nutribullet Extractor Blade on to the top of the cup. Invert the cup, press it down into the Nutribullet Power Base and twist it into place. Blast the mixture until it is really smooth (20 or so seconds). **Enjoy!**

Raspberry Dictator

Ingredients

1 Cup/Handful of Broccoli Florets (40 grams or 1½ oz)
1 Cup/Handful of Spinach (40 grams or 1½ oz)
1 Cup of Raspberries (120 grams or 4 oz)
1 Cup of Blackberries (120 grams or 4 oz)
200 ml / 7 fl oz of Almond Milk (Unsweetened)

Protein 6g, Fat 4g, Carb 14g, Fibre 17g, 162 Kcals

Preparation

Put all the solid ingredients into the Tall Cup and press them down below the Max Line. Add the fluid base to fill the cup up to the Max Line. Screw the Nutribullet Extractor Blade on to the top of the cup. Invert the cup, press it down into the Nutribullet Power Base and twist it into place. Blast the mixture until it is really smooth (20 or so seconds). **Enjoy!**

Blueberry embraces Goji

Ingredients

1 Cup/Handful of Spinach (40 grams or 1½ oz)
1 Cup/Handful of Broccoli Florets (40 grams or 1½ oz)
1 Cup of Blueberries (120 grams or 4 oz)
½ Cup of Goji Berries Dried (40 grams or 1½ oz)
200 ml / 7 fl oz of Water

Protein 9g, Fat 1g, Carb 39g, Fibre 7g, 219 Kcals

Preparation

Put all the solid ingredients into the Tall Cup and press them down below the Max Line. Add the fluid base to fill the cup up to the Max Line. Screw the Nutribullet Extractor Blade on to the top of the cup. Invert the cup, press it down into the Nutribullet Power Base and twist it into place. Blast the mixture until it is really smooth (20 or so seconds). **Enjoy!**

Apricot Chorus

Ingredients

2 Cups/Handfuls of Broccoli Florets (80 grams or 3 oz)
2 Cups of Apricot halves (240 grams or 8 oz)
200 ml / 7 fl oz of Dairy Milk Whole

Protein 12g, Fat 8g, Carb 35g, Fibre 7g, 270 Kcals

Preparation

Put all the solid ingredients into the Tall Cup and press them down below the Max Line. Add the fluid base to fill the cup up to the Max Line. Screw the Nutribullet Extractor Blade on to the top of the cup. Invert the cup, press it down into the Nutribullet Power Base and twist it into place. Blast the mixture until it is really smooth (20 or so seconds). **Enjoy!**

Chard and Guava Infusion

Ingredients

1 Cup/Handful of Swiss Chard (40 grams or 1½ oz)
1 Cup/Handful of Broccoli Florets (40 grams or 1½ oz)
1 Cup of Papaya (120 grams or 4 oz)
1 Cup of Guava (120 grams or 4 oz)
200 ml / 7 fl oz of Water

Protein 6g, Fat 2g, Carb 24g, Fibre 10g, 154 Kcals

Preparation

Put all the solid ingredients into the Tall Cup and press them down below the Max Line. Add the fluid base to fill the cup up to the Max Line. Screw the Nutribullet Extractor Blade on to the top of the cup. Invert the cup, press it down into the Nutribullet Power Base and twist it into place. Blast the mixture until it is really smooth (20 or so seconds). **Enjoy!**

Blueberry hugs Beetroot

Ingredients

2 Cups/Handfuls of Broccoli Florets (80 grams or 3 oz)
1 Cup of Blueberries (120 grams or 4 oz)
1 Cup of diced Beetroot (120 grams or 4 oz)
200 ml / 7 fl oz of Dairy Milk Whole

Protein 11g, Fat 8g, Carb 35g, Fibre 8g, 275 Kcals

Preparation

Put all the solid ingredients into the Tall Cup and press them down below the Max Line. Add the fluid base to fill the cup up to the Max Line. Screw the Nutribullet Extractor Blade on to the top of the cup. Invert the cup, press it down into the Nutribullet Power Base and twist it into place. Blast the mixture until it is really smooth (20 or so seconds). *Enjoy!*

Spinach Treat

Ingredients

1 Cup/Handful of Swiss Chard (40 grams or 1½ oz)
1 Cup/Handful of Spinach (40 grams or 1½ oz)
½ Cup of Goji Berries Dried (40 grams or 1½ oz)
1 Cup of sliced Tomato (120 grams or 4 oz)
200 ml / 7 fl oz of Water

Protein 9g, Fat 1g, Carb 27g, Fibre 5g, 166 Kcals

Preparation

Put all the solid ingredients into the Tall Cup and press them down below the Max Line. Add the fluid base to fill the cup up to the Max Line. Screw the Nutribullet Extractor Blade on to the top of the cup. Invert the cup, press it down into the Nutribullet Power Base and twist it into place. Blast the mixture until it is really smooth (20 or so seconds). *Enjoy!*

Carrot Opera

Ingredients

1 Cup/Handful of Broccoli Florets (40 grams or 1½ oz)
1 Cup/Handful of Swiss Chard (40 grams or 1½ oz)
1 Cup of Raspberries (120 grams or 4 oz)
1 Cup of sliced Carrots (120 grams or 4 oz)
200 ml / 7 fl oz of Almond Milk (Unsweetened)

Protein 5g, Fat 3g, Carb 17g, Fibre 14g, 158 Kcals

Preparation

Put all the solid ingredients into the Tall Cup and press them down below the Max Line. Add the fluid base to fill the cup up to the Max Line. Screw the Nutribullet Extractor Blade on to the top of the cup. Invert the cup, press it down into the Nutribullet Power Base and twist it into place. Blast the mixture until it is really smooth (20 or so seconds). **Enjoy!**

Spinach partners Avocado

Ingredients

2 Cups/Handfuls of Spinach (80 grams or 3 oz)
1 small Avocado (stoned and peeled) (120 grams or 4 oz)
1 Cup of diced Beetroot (120 grams or 4 oz)
200 ml / 7 fl oz of Dairy Milk Whole

Protein 13g, Fat 25g, Carb 21g, Fibre 13g, 390 Kcals

Preparation

Put all the solid ingredients into the Tall Cup and press them down below the Max Line. Add the fluid base to fill the cup up to the Max Line. Screw the Nutribullet Extractor Blade on to the top of the cup. Invert the cup, press it down into the Nutribullet Power Base and twist it into place. Blast the mixture until it is really smooth (20 or so seconds). **Enjoy!**

Broccoli and Guava Explosion

Ingredients

2 Cups/Handfuls of Broccoli Florets (80 grams or 3 oz)
1 Cup of Guava (120 grams or 4 oz)
1 Cup of sliced Tomato (120 grams or 4 oz)
200 ml / 7 fl oz of Water

Protein 6g, Fat 2g, Carb 17g, Fibre 10g, 130 Kcals

Preparation

Put all the solid ingredients into the Tall Cup and press them down below the Max Line. Add the fluid base to fill the cup up to the Max Line. Screw the Nutribullet Extractor Blade on to the top of the cup. Invert the cup, press it down into the Nutribullet Power Base and twist it into place. Blast the mixture until it is really smooth (20 or so seconds). **Enjoy!**

Broccoli Soother

Ingredients

1 Cup/Handful of Broccoli Florets (40 grams or 1½ oz)
1 Cup/Handful of Spinach (40 grams or 1½ oz)
1 Cup of Apricot halves (120 grams or 4 oz)
1 Cup of sliced Carrots (120 grams or 4 oz)
200 ml / 7 fl oz of Almond Milk (Unsweetened)

Protein 6g, Fat 3g, Carb 21g, Fibre 8g, 155 Kcals

Preparation

Put all the solid ingredients into the Tall Cup and press them down below the Max Line. Add the fluid base to fill the cup up to the Max Line. Screw the Nutribullet Extractor Blade on to the top of the cup. Invert the cup, press it down into the Nutribullet Power Base and twist it into place. Blast the mixture until it is really smooth (20 or so seconds). **Enjoy!**

Chard and Blackberry Dream

Ingredients

1 Cup/Handful of Swiss Chard (40 grams or 1½ oz)
1 Cup/Handful of Broccoli Florets (40 grams or 1½ oz)
1 Cup of Blackberries (120 grams or 4 oz)
1 Cup of sliced Tomato (120 grams or 4 oz)
200 ml / 7 fl oz of Dairy Milk Whole

Protein 11g, Fat 8g, Carb 20g, Fibre 9g, 222 Kcals

Preparation

Put all the solid ingredients into the Tall Cup and press them down below the Max Line. Add the fluid base to fill the cup up to the Max Line. Screw the Nutribullet Extractor Blade on to the top of the cup. Invert the cup, press it down into the Nutribullet Power Base and twist it into place. Blast the mixture until it is really smooth (20 or so seconds). **Enjoy!**

Papaya Extravaganza

Ingredients

1 Cup/Handful of Spinach (40 grams or 1½ oz)
1 Cup/Handful of Swiss Chard (40 grams or 1½ oz)
1 Cup of Papaya (120 grams or 4 oz)
1 Cup of sliced Carrots (120 grams or 4 oz)
200 ml / 7 fl oz of Water

Protein 4g, Fat 0.8g, Carb 20g, Fibre 7g, 117 Kcals

Preparation

Put all the solid ingredients into the Tall Cup and press them down below the Max Line. Add the fluid base to fill the cup up to the Max Line. Screw the Nutribullet Extractor Blade on to the top of the cup. Invert the cup, press it down into the Nutribullet Power Base and twist it into place. Blast the mixture until it is really smooth (20 or so seconds). **Enjoy!**

Broccoli and Goji Supermodel

Ingredients

2 Cups/Handfuls of Broccoli Florets (80 grams or 3 oz)
½ Cup of Goji Berries Dried (40 grams or 1½ oz)
1 Cup of diced Beetroot (120 grams or 4 oz)
200 ml / 7 fl oz of Almond Milk (Unsweetened)

Protein 11g, Fat 3g, Carb 34g, Fibre 8g, 233 Kcals

Preparation

Put all the solid ingredients into the Tall Cup and press them down below the Max Line. Add the fluid base to fill the cup up to the Max Line. Screw the Nutribullet Extractor Blade on to the top of the cup. Invert the cup, press it down into the Nutribullet Power Base and twist it into place. Blast the mixture until it is really smooth (20 or so seconds). *Enjoy!*

Blackberry Fantasy

Ingredients

1 Cup/Handful of Spinach (40 grams or 1½ oz)
1 Cup/Handful of Broccoli Florets (40 grams or 1½ oz)
1 Cup of Blackberries (120 grams or 4 oz)
1 Cup of diced Beetroot (120 grams or 4 oz)
200 ml / 7 fl oz of Dairy Milk Whole

Protein 12g, Fat 8g, Carb 25g, Fibre 12g, 254 Kcals

Preparation

Put all the solid ingredients into the Tall Cup and press them down below the Max Line. Add the fluid base to fill the cup up to the Max Line. Screw the Nutribullet Extractor Blade on to the top of the cup. Invert the cup, press it down into the Nutribullet Power Base and twist it into place. Blast the mixture until it is really smooth (20 or so seconds). *Enjoy!*

Green Cabbage hugs Broccoli

Ingredients

1 Cup/Handful of Green Cabbage (40 grams or 1½ oz)
1 Cup/Handful of Broccoli Florets (40 grams or 1½ oz)
2 Cups of Blackberries (240 grams or 8 oz)
22 grams or ¾ oz of Flax Seeds
200 ml / 7 fl oz of Almond Milk (Unsweetened)

Protein 10g, Fat 13g, Carb 14g, Fibre 22g, 270 Kcals

Preparation

Place the nuts or seeds into the Tall Cup. Screw the Nutribullet Extractor Blade on to the top of the cup. Invert the cup, press it down into the Nutribullet Power Base and twist it into place. Blast them for 30 seconds. Put the rest of the solid ingredients into the cup and press them down below the Max Line. Add the fluid base to fill the cup up to the Max Line. Screw the Nutribullet Extractor Blade on to the top of the cup. Invert the cup, press it down into the Nutribullet Power Base and twist it into place. Blast the mixture until it is really smooth (20 or so seconds). ***Enjoy!***

Red Cabbage goes Cranberry

Ingredients

1 Cup/Handful of Red or White Cabbage (40 grams or 1½ oz)
1 Cup/Handful of Spinach (40 grams or 1½ oz)
1 Cup of Cranberries (120 grams or 4 oz)
1 Cup of Blueberries (120 grams or 4 oz)
30 grams or 1 oz of Almonds
200 ml / 7 fl oz of Water

Protein 9g, Fat 17g, Carb 28g, Fibre 13g, 322 Kcals

Preparation

Place the nuts or seeds into the Tall Cup. Screw the Nutribullet Extractor Blade on to the top of the cup. Invert the cup, press it down into the Nutribullet Power Base and twist it into place. Blast them for 30 seconds. Put the rest of the solid ingredients into the cup and press them down below the Max Line. Add the fluid base to fill the cup up to the Max Line. Screw the Nutribullet Extractor Blade on to the top of the cup. Invert the cup, press it down into the Nutribullet Power Base and twist it into place. Blast the mixture until it is really smooth (20 or so seconds). ***Enjoy!***

Strawberry Wonder

Ingredients

2 Cups/Handfuls of Red or White Cabbage (80 grams or 3 oz)
1 Cup of Strawberries (120 grams or 4 oz)
1 Cup of Raspberries (120 grams or 4 oz)
22 grams or ¾ oz of Sunflower Seeds Hulled
200 ml / 7 fl oz of Water

Protein 8g, Fat 12g, Carb 20g, Fibre 13g, 239 Kcals

Preparation

Place the nuts or seeds into the Tall Cup. Screw the Nutribullet Extractor Blade on to the top of the cup. Invert the cup, press it down into the Nutribullet Power Base and twist it into place. Blast them for 30 seconds. Put the rest of the solid ingredients into the cup and press them down below the Max Line. Add the fluid base to fill the cup up to the Max Line. Screw the Nutribullet Extractor Blade on to the top of the cup. Invert the cup, press it down into the Nutribullet Power Base and twist it into place. Blast the mixture until it is really smooth (20 or so seconds). **Enjoy!**

Blackberry and Walnut Utopia

Ingredients

1 Cup/Handful of Broccoli Florets (40 grams or 1½ oz)
1 Cup/Handful of Spinach (40 grams or 1½ oz)
1 Cup of Blackberries (120 grams or 4 oz)
1 Cup of Plum halves (120 grams or 4 oz)
30 grams or 1 oz of Walnuts
200 ml / 7 fl oz of Almond Milk (Unsweetened)

Protein 10g, Fat 23g, Carb 22g, Fibre 13g, 351 Kcals

Preparation

Place the nuts or seeds into the Tall Cup. Screw the Nutribullet Extractor Blade on to the top of the cup. Invert the cup, press it down into the Nutribullet Power Base and twist it into place. Blast them for 30 seconds. Put the rest of the solid ingredients into the cup and press them down below the Max Line. Add the fluid base to fill the cup up to the Max Line. Screw the Nutribullet Extractor Blade on to the top of the cup. Invert the cup, press it down into the Nutribullet Power Base and twist it into place. Blast the mixture until it is really smooth (20 or so seconds). **Enjoy!**

Papaya embraces Pecan

Ingredients

1 Cup/Handful of Green Cabbage (40 grams or 1½ oz)
1 Cup/Handful of Red or White Cabbage (40 grams or 1½ oz)
1 Cup of Papaya (120 grams or 4 oz)
½ Cup of Goji Berries Dried (40 grams or 1½ oz)
30 grams or 1 oz of Pecans
200 ml / 7 fl oz of Almond Milk (Unsweetened)

Protein 11g, Fat 25g, Carb 39g, Fibre 9g, 435 Kcals

Preparation

Place the nuts or seeds into the Tall Cup. Screw the Nutribullet Extractor Blade on to the top of the cup. Invert the cup, press it down into the Nutribullet Power Base and twist it into place. Blast them for 30 seconds. Put the rest of the solid ingredients into the cup and press them down below the Max Line. Add the fluid base to fill the cup up to the Max Line. Screw the Nutribullet Extractor Blade on to the top of the cup. Invert the cup, press it down into the Nutribullet Power Base and twist it into place. Blast the mixture until it is really smooth (20 or so seconds). **Enjoy!**

Broccoli Opera

Ingredients

1 Cup/Handful of Broccoli Florets (40 grams or 1½ oz)
1 Cup/Handful of Green Cabbage (40 grams or 1½ oz)
2 Cups of Guava (240 grams or 8 oz)
22 grams or ¾ oz of Sesame Seeds Hulled
200 ml / 7 fl oz of Water

Protein 12g, Fat 15g, Carb 25g, Fibre 17g, 318 Kcals

Preparation

Place the nuts or seeds into the Tall Cup. Screw the Nutribullet Extractor Blade on to the top of the cup. Invert the cup, press it down into the Nutribullet Power Base and twist it into place. Blast them for 30 seconds. Put the rest of the solid ingredients into the cup and press them down below the Max Line. Add the fluid base to fill the cup up to the Max Line. Screw the Nutribullet Extractor Blade on to the top of the cup. Invert the cup, press it down into the Nutribullet Power Base and twist it into place. Blast the mixture until it is really smooth (20 or so seconds). **Enjoy!**

Red Cabbage and Apple Surprise

Ingredients

1 Cup/Handful of Red or White Cabbage (40 grams or 1½ oz)
1 Cup/Handful of Spinach (40 grams or 1½ oz)
1 small Apple (cored) (120 grams or 4 oz)
1 Cup of Guava (120 grams or 4 oz)
30 grams or 1 oz of Hazelnuts
200 ml / 7 fl oz of Almond Milk (Unsweetened)

Protein 10g, Fat 22g, Carb 29g, Fibre 15g, 379 Kcals

Preparation

Place the nuts or seeds into the Tall Cup. Screw the Nutribullet Extractor Blade on to the top of the cup. Invert the cup, press it down into the Nutribullet Power Base and twist it into place. Blast them for 30 seconds. Put the rest of the solid ingredients into the cup and press them down below the Max Line. Add the fluid base to fill the cup up to the Max Line. Screw the Nutribullet Extractor Blade on to the top of the cup. Invert the cup, press it down into the Nutribullet Power Base and twist it into place. Blast the mixture until it is really smooth (20 or so seconds). *Enjoy!*

Raspberry joins Sunflower

Ingredients

2 Cups/Handfuls of Spinach (80 grams or 3 oz)
2 Cups of Raspberries (240 grams or 8 oz)
22 grams or ¾ oz of Sunflower Seeds Hulled
200 ml / 7 fl oz of Water

Protein 10g, Fat 12g, Carb 17g, Fibre 19g, 257 Kcals

Preparation

Place the nuts or seeds into the Tall Cup. Screw the Nutribullet Extractor Blade on to the top of the cup. Invert the cup, press it down into the Nutribullet Power Base and twist it into place. Blast them for 30 seconds. Put the rest of the solid ingredients into the cup and press them down below the Max Line. Add the fluid base to fill the cup up to the Max Line. Screw the Nutribullet Extractor Blade on to the top of the cup. Invert the cup, press it down into the Nutribullet Power Base and twist it into place. Blast the mixture until it is really smooth (20 or so seconds). *Enjoy!*

Pear meets Sesame

Ingredients

1 Cup/Handful of Broccoli Florets (40 grams or 1½ oz)
1 Cup/Handful of Green Cabbage (40 grams or 1½ oz)
1 Cup of Prunes (stoned) (120 grams or 4 oz)
1 small Pear (cored) (120 grams or 4 oz)
22 grams or ¾ oz of Sesame Seeds Hulled
200 ml / 7 fl oz of Almond Milk (Unsweetened)

Protein 8g, Fat 17g, Carb 23g, Fibre 11g, 254 Kcals

Preparation

Place the nuts or seeds into the Tall Cup. Screw the Nutribullet Extractor Blade on to the top of the cup. Invert the cup, press it down into the Nutribullet Power Base and twist it into place. Blast them for 30 seconds. Put the rest of the solid ingredients into the cup and press them down below the Max Line. Add the fluid base to fill the cup up to the Max Line. Screw the Nutribullet Extractor Blade on to the top of the cup. Invert the cup, press it down into the Nutribullet Power Base and twist it into place. Blast the mixture until it is really smooth (20 or so seconds). ***Enjoy!***

Cherry Heaven

Ingredients

1 Cup/Handful of Red or White Cabbage (40 grams or 1½ oz)
1 Cup/Handful of Spinach (40 grams or 1½ oz)
1 Cup of Cherries (stoned) (120 grams or 4 oz)
1 Cup of Raspberries (120 grams or 4 oz)
30 grams or 1 oz of Walnuts
200 ml / 7 fl oz of Water

Protein 9g, Fat 21g, Carb 28g, Fibre 14g, 355 Kcals

Preparation

Place the nuts or seeds into the Tall Cup. Screw the Nutribullet Extractor Blade on to the top of the cup. Invert the cup, press it down into the Nutribullet Power Base and twist it into place. Blast them for 30 seconds. Put the rest of the solid ingredients into the cup and press them down below the Max Line. Add the fluid base to fill the cup up to the Max Line. Screw the Nutribullet Extractor Blade on to the top of the cup. Invert the cup, press it down into the Nutribullet Power Base and twist it into place. Blast the mixture until it is really smooth (20 or so seconds). ***Enjoy!***

Apple befriends Flax

Ingredients

1 Cup/Handful of Green Cabbage (40 grams or 1½ oz)
1 Cup/Handful of Spinach (40 grams or 1½ oz)
2 small Apples (cored) (240 grams or 8 oz)
22 grams or ¾ oz of Flax Seeds
200 ml / 7 fl oz of Almond Milk (Unsweetened)

Protein 7g, Fat 12g, Carb 30g, Fibre 14g, 287 Kcals

Preparation

Place the nuts or seeds into the Tall Cup. Screw the Nutribullet Extractor Blade on to the top of the cup. Invert the cup, press it down into the Nutribullet Power Base and twist it into place. Blast them for 30 seconds. Put the rest of the solid ingredients into the cup and press them down below the Max Line. Add the fluid base to fill the cup up to the Max Line. Screw the Nutribullet Extractor Blade on to the top of the cup. Invert the cup, press it down into the Nutribullet Power Base and twist it into place. Blast the mixture until it is really smooth (20 or so seconds). **Enjoy!**

Papaya Concerto

Ingredients

2 Cups/Handfuls of Red or White Cabbage (80 grams or 3 oz)
1 Cup of Plum halves (120 grams or 4 oz)
1 Cup of Papaya (120 grams or 4 oz)
30 grams or 1 oz of Pecans
200 ml / 7 fl oz of Water

Protein 5g, Fat 22g, Carb 28g, Fibre 8g, 338 Kcals

Preparation

Place the nuts or seeds into the Tall Cup. Screw the Nutribullet Extractor Blade on to the top of the cup. Invert the cup, press it down into the Nutribullet Power Base and twist it into place. Blast them for 30 seconds. Put the rest of the solid ingredients into the cup and press them down below the Max Line. Add the fluid base to fill the cup up to the Max Line. Screw the Nutribullet Extractor Blade on to the top of the cup. Invert the cup, press it down into the Nutribullet Power Base and twist it into place. Blast the mixture until it is really smooth (20 or so seconds). **Enjoy!**

Red Cabbage and Cranberry Sunshine

Ingredients

1 Cup/Handful of Broccoli Florets (40 grams or 1½ oz)
1 Cup/Handful of Red or White Cabbage (40 grams or 1½ oz)
1 Cup of Cranberries (120 grams or 4 oz)
1 Cup of Prunes (stoned) (120 grams or 4 oz)
30 grams or 1 oz of Almonds
200 ml / 7 fl oz of Almond Milk (Unsweetened)

Protein 10g, Fat 20g, Carb 19g, Fibre 14g, 289 Kcals

Preparation

Place the nuts or seeds into the Tall Cup. Screw the Nutribullet Extractor Blade on to the top of the cup. Invert the cup, press it down into the Nutribullet Power Base and twist it into place. Blast them for 30 seconds. Put the rest of the solid ingredients into the cup and press them down below the Max Line. Add the fluid base to fill the cup up to the Max Line. Screw the Nutribullet Extractor Blade on to the top of the cup. Invert the cup, press it down into the Nutribullet Power Base and twist it into place. Blast the mixture until it is really smooth (20 or so seconds). **Enjoy!**

Goji Delivered

Ingredients

1 Cup/Handful of Green Cabbage (40 grams or 1½ oz)
1 Cup/Handful of Spinach (40 grams or 1½ oz)
1 small Pear (cored) (120 grams or 4 oz)
½ Cup of Goji Berries Dried (40 grams or 1½ oz)
30 grams or 1 oz of Hazelnuts
200 ml / 7 fl oz of Water

Protein 12g, Fat 19g, Carb 43g, Fibre 10g, 404 Kcals

Preparation

Place the nuts or seeds into the Tall Cup. Screw the Nutribullet Extractor Blade on to the top of the cup. Invert the cup, press it down into the Nutribullet Power Base and twist it into place. Blast them for 30 seconds. Put the rest of the solid ingredients into the cup and press them down below the Max Line. Add the fluid base to fill the cup up to the Max Line. Screw the Nutribullet Extractor Blade on to the top of the cup. Invert the cup, press it down into the Nutribullet Power Base and twist it into place. Blast the mixture until it is really smooth (20 or so seconds). **Enjoy!**

Blueberry Miracle

Ingredients

1 Cup/Handful of Broccoli Florets (40 grams or 1½ oz)
1 Cup/Handful of Red or White Cabbage (40 grams or 1½ oz)
1 Cup of Blueberries (120 grams or 4 oz)
1 Cup of Strawberries (120 grams or 4 oz)
22 grams or ¾ oz of Flax Seeds
200 ml / 7 fl oz of Water

Protein 7g, Fat 10g, Carb 25g, Fibre 13g, 250 Kcals

Preparation

Place the nuts or seeds into the Tall Cup. Screw the Nutribullet Extractor Blade on to the top of the cup. Invert the cup, press it down into the Nutribullet Power Base and twist it into place. Blast them for 30 seconds. Put the rest of the solid ingredients into the cup and press them down below the Max Line. Add the fluid base to fill the cup up to the Max Line. Screw the Nutribullet Extractor Blade on to the top of the cup. Invert the cup, press it down into the Nutribullet Power Base and twist it into place. Blast the mixture until it is really smooth (20 or so seconds). **Enjoy!**

Anti Oxidizing Smoothies
All ingredients are high in antioxidants

Spinach and Cherry Morning

Ingredients

1 Cup/Handful of Red or White Cabbage (40 grams or 1½ oz)
1 Cup/Handful of Spinach (40 grams or 1½ oz)
1 Cup of Cherries (stoned) (120 grams or 4 oz)
1 Cup of Blackberries (120 grams or 4 oz)
200 ml / 7 fl oz of Water

Protein 5g, Fat 1g, Carb 25g, Fibre 11g, 148 Kcals

Preparation

Put all the solid ingredients into the Tall Cup and press them down below the Max Line. Add the fluid base to fill the cup up to the Max Line. Screw the Nutribullet Extractor Blade on to the top of the cup. Invert the cup, press it down into the Nutribullet Power Base and twist it into place. Blast the mixture until it is really smooth (20 or so seconds). **Enjoy!**

Papaya Opera

Ingredients

1 Cup/Handful of Broccoli Florets (40 grams or 1½ oz)
1 Cup/Handful of Green Cabbage (40 grams or 1½ oz)
½ Cup of Goji Berries Dried (40 grams or 1½ oz)
1 Cup of Papaya (120 grams or 4 oz)
200 ml / 7 fl oz of Almond Milk (Unsweetened)

Protein 9g, Fat 3g, Carb 37g, Fibre 7g, 229 Kcals

Preparation

Put all the solid ingredients into the Tall Cup and press them down below the Max Line. Add the fluid base to fill the cup up to the Max Line. Screw the Nutribullet Extractor Blade on to the top of the cup. Invert the cup, press it down into the Nutribullet Power Base and twist it into place. Blast the mixture until it is really smooth (20 or so seconds). **Enjoy!**

Spinach Invigorator

Ingredients

1 Cup/Handful of Broccoli Florets (40 grams or 1½ oz)
1 Cup/Handful of Spinach (40 grams or 1½ oz)
2 Cups of Prunes (stoned) (240 grams or 8 oz)
200 ml / 7 fl oz of Almond Milk (Unsweetened)

Protein 5g, Fat 7g, Carb 10g, Fibre 9g, 58 Kcals

Preparation

Put all the solid ingredients into the Tall Cup and press them down below the Max Line. Add the fluid base to fill the cup up to the Max Line. Screw the Nutribullet Extractor Blade on to the top of the cup. Invert the cup, press it down into the Nutribullet Power Base and twist it into place. Blast the mixture until it is really smooth (20 or so seconds). **Enjoy!**

Blueberry Ensemble

Ingredients

1 Cup/Handful of Red or White Cabbage (40 grams or 1½ oz)
1 Cup/Handful of Green Cabbage (40 grams or 1½ oz)
1 Cup of Raspberries (120 grams or 4 oz)
1 Cup of Blueberries (120 grams or 4 oz)
200 ml / 7 fl oz of Water

Protein 3g, Fat 1g, Carb 24g, Fibre 13g, 153 Kcals

Preparation

Put all the solid ingredients into the Tall Cup and press them down below the Max Line. Add the fluid base to fill the cup up to the Max Line. Screw the Nutribullet Extractor Blade on to the top of the cup. Invert the cup, press it down into the Nutribullet Power Base and twist it into place. Blast the mixture until it is really smooth (20 or so seconds). **Enjoy!**

Prune Symphony

Ingredients

1 Cup/Handful of Green Cabbage (40 grams or 1½ oz)
1 Cup/Handful of Spinach (40 grams or 1½ oz)
1 Cup of Prunes (stoned) (120 grams or 4 oz)
1 Cup of Cranberries (120 grams or 4 oz)
200 ml / 7 fl oz of Almond Milk (Unsweetened)

Protein 4g, Fat 5g, Carb 15g, Fibre 11g, 105 Kcals

Preparation

Put all the solid ingredients into the Tall Cup and press them down below the Max Line. Add the fluid base to fill the cup up to the Max Line. Screw the Nutribullet Extractor Blade on to the top of the cup. Invert the cup, press it down into the Nutribullet Power Base and twist it into place. Blast the mixture until it is really smooth (20 or so seconds). **Enjoy!**

Pineapple goes Sesame

Ingredients

2 Cups/Handfuls of Broccoli Florets (80 grams or 3 oz)
2 Cups of Pineapple chunks (240 grams or 8 oz)
22 grams or ¾ oz of Sesame Seeds Hulled
200 ml / 7 fl oz of Water

Protein 8g, Fat 13g, Carb 32g, Fibre 7g, 278 Kcals

Preparation

Place the nuts or seeds into the Tall Cup. Screw the Nutribullet Extractor Blade on to the top of the cup. Invert the cup, press it down into the Nutribullet Power Base and twist it into place. Blast them for 30 seconds. Put the rest of the solid ingredients into the cup and press them down below the Max Line. Add the fluid base to fill the cup up to the Max Line. Screw the Nutribullet Extractor Blade on to the top of the cup. Invert the cup, press it down into the Nutribullet Power Base and twist it into place. Blast the mixture until it is really smooth (20 or so seconds). *Enjoy!*

Green Cabbage and Apple Vision

Ingredients

1 Cup/Handful of Green Cabbage (40 grams or 1½ oz)
1 Cup/Handful of Fennel (40 grams or 1½ oz)
2 small Apples (cored) (240 grams or 8 oz)
30 grams or 1 oz of Brazil nuts
200 ml / 7 fl oz of Water

Protein 6g, Fat 21g, Carb 32g, Fibre 10g, 344 Kcals

Preparation

Place the nuts or seeds into the Tall Cup. Screw the Nutribullet Extractor Blade on to the top of the cup. Invert the cup, press it down into the Nutribullet Power Base and twist it into place. Blast them for 30 seconds. Put the rest of the solid ingredients into the cup and press them down below the Max Line. Add the fluid base to fill the cup up to the Max Line. Screw the Nutribullet Extractor Blade on to the top of the cup. Invert the cup, press it down into the Nutribullet Power Base and twist it into place. Blast the mixture until it is really smooth (20 or so seconds). *Enjoy!*

Watercress embraces Apple

Ingredients

1 Cup/Handful of Red or White Cabbage (40 grams or 1½ oz)
1 Cup/Handful of Watercress (40 grams or 1½ oz)
1 small Apple (cored) (120 grams or 4 oz)
1 Cup of Pineapple chunks (120 grams or 4 oz)
22 grams or ¾ oz of Sesame Seeds Hulled
200 ml / 7 fl oz of Water

Protein 6g, Fat 13g, Carb 30g, Fibre 7g, 270 Kcals

Preparation

Place the nuts or seeds into the Tall Cup. Screw the Nutribullet Extractor Blade on to the top of the cup. Invert the cup, press it down into the Nutribullet Power Base and twist it into place. Blast them for 30 seconds. Put the rest of the solid ingredients into the cup and press them down below the Max Line. Add the fluid base to fill the cup up to the Max Line. Screw the Nutribullet Extractor Blade on to the top of the cup. Invert the cup, press it down into the Nutribullet Power Base and twist it into place. Blast the mixture until it is really smooth (20 or so seconds). *Enjoy!*

Brazil Salad

Ingredients

2 Cups/Handfuls of Green Cabbage (80 grams or 3 oz)
2 Cups of Grapefruit segments (240 grams or 8 oz)
30 grams or 1 oz of Brazil nuts
200 ml / 7 fl oz of Water

Protein 7g, Fat 20g, Carb 21g, Fibre 7g, 294 Kcals

Preparation

Place the nuts or seeds into the Tall Cup. Screw the Nutribullet Extractor Blade on to the top of the cup. Invert the cup, press it down into the Nutribullet Power Base and twist it into place. Blast them for 30 seconds. Put the rest of the solid ingredients into the cup and press them down below the Max Line. Add the fluid base to fill the cup up to the Max Line. Screw the Nutribullet Extractor Blade on to the top of the cup. Invert the cup, press it down into the Nutribullet Power Base and twist it into place. Blast the mixture until it is really smooth (20 or so seconds). *Enjoy!*

Avocado hugs Grapefruit

Ingredients

1 Cup/Handful of Broccoli Florets (40 grams or 1½ oz)
1 Cup/Handful of Red or White Cabbage (40 grams or 1½ oz)
1 small Avocado (stoned and peeled) (120 grams or 4 oz)
1 Cup of Grapefruit segments (120 grams or 4 oz)
22 grams or ¾ oz of Sesame Seeds Hulled
200 ml / 7 fl oz of Water

Protein 9g, Fat 31g, Carb 15g, Fibre 13g, 387 Kcals

Preparation

Place the nuts or seeds into the Tall Cup. Screw the Nutribullet Extractor Blade on to the top of the cup. Invert the cup, press it down into the Nutribullet Power Base and twist it into place. Blast them for 30 seconds. Put the rest of the solid ingredients into the cup and press them down below the Max Line. Add the fluid base to fill the cup up to the Max Line. Screw the Nutribullet Extractor Blade on to the top of the cup. Invert the cup, press it down into the Nutribullet Power Base and twist it into place. Blast the mixture until it is really smooth (20 or so seconds). **Enjoy!**

Watercress meets Brazil

Ingredients

2 Cups/Handfuls of Watercress (80 grams or 3 oz)
1 small Avocado (stoned and peeled) (120 grams or 4 oz)
1 Cup of Grapefruit segments (120 grams or 4 oz)
30 grams or 1 oz of Brazil nuts
200 ml / 7 fl oz of Water

Protein 9g, Fat 38g, Carb 12g, Fibre 12g, 436 Kcals

Preparation

Place the nuts or seeds into the Tall Cup. Screw the Nutribullet Extractor Blade on to the top of the cup. Invert the cup, press it down into the Nutribullet Power Base and twist it into place. Blast them for 30 seconds. Put the rest of the solid ingredients into the cup and press them down below the Max Line. Add the fluid base to fill the cup up to the Max Line. Screw the Nutribullet Extractor Blade on to the top of the cup. Invert the cup, press it down into the Nutribullet Power Base and twist it into place. Blast the mixture until it is really smooth (20 or so seconds). **Enjoy!**

Broccoli Cocktail

Ingredients

1 Cup/Handful of Green Cabbage (40 grams or 1½ oz)
1 Cup/Handful of Broccoli Florets (40 grams or 1½ oz)
2 Cups of Pineapple chunks (240 grams or 8 oz)
30 grams or 1 oz of Brazil nuts
200 ml / 7 fl oz of Water

Protein 7g, Fat 21g, Carb 32g, Fibre 8g, 341 Kcals

Preparation

Place the nuts or seeds into the Tall Cup. Screw the Nutribullet Extractor Blade on to the top of the cup. Invert the cup, press it down into the Nutribullet Power Base and twist it into place. Blast them for 30 seconds. Put the rest of the solid ingredients into the cup and press them down below the Max Line. Add the fluid base to fill the cup up to the Max Line. Screw the Nutribullet Extractor Blade on to the top of the cup. Invert the cup, press it down into the Nutribullet Power Base and twist it into place. Blast the mixture until it is really smooth (20 or so seconds). **Enjoy!**

Watercress and Apple Kiss

Ingredients

1 Cup/Handful of Fennel (40 grams or 1½ oz)
1 Cup/Handful of Watercress (40 grams or 1½ oz)
1 Cup of Pineapple chunks (120 grams or 4 oz)
1 small Apple (cored) (120 grams or 4 oz)
22 grams or ¾ oz of Sesame Seeds Hulled
200 ml / 7 fl oz of Water

Protein 6g, Fat 13g, Carb 30g, Fibre 8g, 270 Kcals

Preparation

Place the nuts or seeds into the Tall Cup. Screw the Nutribullet Extractor Blade on to the top of the cup. Invert the cup, press it down into the Nutribullet Power Base and twist it into place. Blast them for 30 seconds. Put the rest of the solid ingredients into the cup and press them down below the Max Line. Add the fluid base to fill the cup up to the Max Line. Screw the Nutribullet Extractor Blade on to the top of the cup. Invert the cup, press it down into the Nutribullet Power Base and twist it into place. Blast the mixture until it is really smooth (20 or so seconds). **Enjoy!**

Green Cabbage and Grapefruit Mist

Ingredients

1 Cup/Handful of Green Cabbage (40 grams or 1½ oz)
1 Cup/Handful of Red or White Cabbage (40 grams or 1½ oz)
1 Cup of Grapefruit segments (120 grams or 4 oz)
1 small Avocado (stoned and peeled) (120 grams or 4 oz)
30 grams or 1 oz of Brazil nuts
200 ml / 7 fl oz of Water

Protein 9g, Fat 38g, Carb 15g, Fibre 13g, 450 Kcals

Preparation

Place the nuts or seeds into the Tall Cup. Screw the Nutribullet Extractor Blade on to the top of the cup. Invert the cup, press it down into the Nutribullet Power Base and twist it into place. Blast them for 30 seconds. Put the rest of the solid ingredients into the cup and press them down below the Max Line. Add the fluid base to fill the cup up to the Max Line. Screw the Nutribullet Extractor Blade on to the top of the cup. Invert the cup, press it down into the Nutribullet Power Base and twist it into place. Blast the mixture until it is really smooth (20 or so seconds). **Enjoy!**

Fennel joins Apple

Ingredients

1 Cup/Handful of Broccoli Florets (40 grams or 1½ oz)
1 Cup/Handful of Fennel (40 grams or 1½ oz)
1 Cup of Pineapple chunks (120 grams or 4 oz)
1 small Apple (cored) (120 grams or 4 oz)
22 grams or ¾ oz of Sesame Seeds Hulled
200 ml / 7 fl oz of Water

Protein 7g, Fat 13g, Carb 31g, Fibre 9g, 279 Kcals

Preparation

Place the nuts or seeds into the Tall Cup. Screw the Nutribullet Extractor Blade on to the top of the cup. Invert the cup, press it down into the Nutribullet Power Base and twist it into place. Blast them for 30 seconds. Put the rest of the solid ingredients into the cup and press them down below the Max Line. Add the fluid base to fill the cup up to the Max Line. Screw the Nutribullet Extractor Blade on to the top of the cup. Invert the cup, press it down into the Nutribullet Power Base and twist it into place. Blast the mixture until it is really smooth (20 or so seconds). **Enjoy!**

Fennel and Pineapple Blockbuster

Ingredients

2 Cups/Handfuls of Fennel (80 grams or 3 oz)
1 Cup of Pineapple chunks (120 grams or 4 oz)
1 Cup of diced Beetroot (120 grams or 4 oz)
22 grams or ¾ oz of Sesame Seeds Hulled
200 ml / 7 fl oz of Water

Protein 8g, Fat 13g, Carb 26g, Fibre 9g, 267 Kcals

Preparation

Place the nuts or seeds into the Tall Cup. Screw the Nutribullet Extractor Blade on to the top of the cup. Invert the cup, press it down into the Nutribullet Power Base and twist it into place. Blast them for 30 seconds. Put the rest of the solid ingredients into the cup and press them down below the Max Line. Add the fluid base to fill the cup up to the Max Line. Screw the Nutribullet Extractor Blade on to the top of the cup. Invert the cup, press it down into the Nutribullet Power Base and twist it into place. Blast the mixture until it is really smooth (20 or so seconds). *Enjoy!*

Avocado Fiesta

Ingredients

1 Cup/Handful of Green Cabbage (40 grams or 1½ oz)
1 Cup/Handful of Watercress (40 grams or 1½ oz)
1 small Avocado (stoned and peeled) (120 grams or 4 oz)
1 Cup of diced Beetroot (120 grams or 4 oz)
30 grams or 1 oz of Brazil nuts
200 ml / 7 fl oz of Water

Protein 10g, Fat 38g, Carb 13g, Fibre 15g, 455 Kcals

Preparation

Place the nuts or seeds into the Tall Cup. Screw the Nutribullet Extractor Blade on to the top of the cup. Invert the cup, press it down into the Nutribullet Power Base and twist it into place. Blast them for 30 seconds. Put the rest of the solid ingredients into the cup and press them down below the Max Line. Add the fluid base to fill the cup up to the Max Line. Screw the Nutribullet Extractor Blade on to the top of the cup. Invert the cup, press it down into the Nutribullet Power Base and twist it into place. Blast the mixture until it is really smooth (20 or so seconds). *Enjoy!*

Avocado partners Pineapple

Ingredients

1 Cup/Handful of Broccoli Florets (40 grams or 1½ oz)
1 Cup/Handful of Watercress (40 grams or 1½ oz)
1 small Avocado (stoned and peeled) (120 grams or 4 oz)
1 Cup of Pineapple chunks (120 grams or 4 oz)
200 ml / 7 fl oz of Water

Protein 5g, Fat 18g, Carb 18g, Fibre 11g, 270 Kcals

Preparation

Put all the solid ingredients into the Tall Cup and press them down below the Max Line. Add the fluid base to fill the cup up to the Max Line. Screw the Nutribullet Extractor Blade on to the top of the cup. Invert the cup, press it down into the Nutribullet Power Base and twist it into place. Blast the mixture until it is really smooth (20 or so seconds). ***Enjoy!***

Red Cabbage meets Apple

Ingredients

1 Cup/Handful of Fennel (40 grams or 1½ oz)
1 Cup/Handful of Red or White Cabbage (40 grams or 1½ oz)
2 small Apples (cored) (240 grams or 8 oz)
200 ml / 7 fl oz of Water

Protein 2g, Fat 0.6g, Carb 31g, Fibre 8g, 149 Kcals

Preparation

Put all the solid ingredients into the Tall Cup and press them down below the Max Line. Add the fluid base to fill the cup up to the Max Line. Screw the Nutribullet Extractor Blade on to the top of the cup. Invert the cup, press it down into the Nutribullet Power Base and twist it into place. Blast the mixture until it is really smooth (20 or so seconds). ***Enjoy!***

Green Cabbage and Apple Sonata

Ingredients

2 Cups/Handfuls of Green Cabbage (80 grams or 3 oz)
1 small Apple (cored) (120 grams or 4 oz)
1 Cup of Grapefruit segments (120 grams or 4 oz)
200 ml / 7 fl oz of Water

Protein 2g, Fat 0.4g, Carb 25g, Fibre 6g, 120 Kcals

Preparation

Put all the solid ingredients into the Tall Cup and press them down below the Max Line. Add the fluid base to fill the cup up to the Max Line. Screw the Nutribullet Extractor Blade on to the top of the cup. Invert the cup, press it down into the Nutribullet Power Base and twist it into place. Blast the mixture until it is really smooth (20 or so seconds). **Enjoy!**

Watercress goes Apple

Ingredients

1 Cup/Handful of Green Cabbage (40 grams or 1½ oz)
1 Cup/Handful of Watercress (40 grams or 1½ oz)
1 small Apple (cored) (120 grams or 4 oz)
1 Cup of Grapefruit segments (120 grams or 4 oz)
200 ml / 7 fl oz of Water

Protein 3g, Fat 0.4g, Carb 24g, Fibre 5g, 115 Kcals

Preparation

Put all the solid ingredients into the Tall Cup and press them down below the Max Line. Add the fluid base to fill the cup up to the Max Line. Screw the Nutribullet Extractor Blade on to the top of the cup. Invert the cup, press it down into the Nutribullet Power Base and twist it into place. Blast the mixture until it is really smooth (20 or so seconds). **Enjoy!**

Watercress Mist

Ingredients

2 Cups/Handfuls of Watercress (80 grams or 3 oz)
2 Cups of Grapefruit segments (240 grams or 8 oz)
200 ml / 7 fl oz of Water

Protein 3g, Fat 0.3g, Carb 17g, Fibre 3g, 85 Kcals

Preparation

Put all the solid ingredients into the Tall Cup and press them down below the Max Line. Add the fluid base to fill the cup up to the Max Line. Screw the Nutribullet Extractor Blade on to the top of the cup. Invert the cup, press it down into the Nutribullet Power Base and twist it into place. Blast the mixture until it is really smooth (20 or so seconds). **Enjoy!**

Fennel and Red Cabbage Dance

Ingredients

1 Cup/Handful of Fennel (40 grams or 1½ oz)
1 Cup/Handful of Red or White Cabbage (40 grams or 1½ oz)
2 Cups of Pineapple chunks (240 grams or 8 oz)
200 ml / 7 fl oz of Water

Protein 2g, Fat 0.4g, Carb 32g, Fibre 5g, 144 Kcals

Preparation

Put all the solid ingredients into the Tall Cup and press them down below the Max Line. Add the fluid base to fill the cup up to the Max Line. Screw the Nutribullet Extractor Blade on to the top of the cup. Invert the cup, press it down into the Nutribullet Power Base and twist it into place. Blast the mixture until it is really smooth (20 or so seconds). **Enjoy!**

Broccoli Royale

Ingredients

2 Cups/Handfuls of Broccoli Florets (80 grams or 3 oz)
2 small Avocado (stoned and peeled) (240 grams or 8 oz)
200 ml / 7 fl oz of Water

Protein 7g, Fat 35g, Carb 8g, Fibre 18g, 411 Kcals

Preparation

Put all the solid ingredients into the Tall Cup and press them down below the Max Line. Add the fluid base to fill the cup up to the Max Line. Screw the Nutribullet Extractor Blade on to the top of the cup. Invert the cup, press it down into the Nutribullet Power Base and twist it into place. Blast the mixture until it is really smooth (20 or so seconds). *Enjoy!*

Broccoli kisses Green Cabbage

Ingredients

1 Cup/Handful of Broccoli Florets (40 grams or 1½ oz)
1 Cup/Handful of Green Cabbage (40 grams or 1½ oz)
1 small Avocado (stoned and peeled) (120 grams or 4 oz)
1 Cup of Pineapple chunks (120 grams or 4 oz)
200 ml / 7 fl oz of Water

Protein 5g, Fat 18g, Carb 19g, Fibre 12g, 275 Kcals

Preparation

Put all the solid ingredients into the Tall Cup and press them down below the Max Line. Add the fluid base to fill the cup up to the Max Line. Screw the Nutribullet Extractor Blade on to the top of the cup. Invert the cup, press it down into the Nutribullet Power Base and twist it into place. Blast the mixture until it is really smooth (20 or so seconds). *Enjoy!*

Broccoli and Rocket Tonic

Ingredients

1 Cup/Handful of Broccoli Florets (40 grams or 1½ oz)
1 Cup/Handful of Rocket/Arugura Lettuce (40 grams or 1½ oz)
1 Cup of Raspberries (120 grams or 4 oz)
1 Cup of Guava (120 grams or 4 oz)
30 grams or 1 oz of Pecans
200 ml / 7 fl oz of Dairy Milk Semi Skimmed

Protein 16g, Fat 27g, Carb 30g, Fibre 19g, 470 Kcals

Preparation

Place the nuts or seeds into the Tall Cup. Screw the Nutribullet Extractor Blade on to the top of the cup. Invert the cup, press it down into the Nutribullet Power Base and twist it into place. Blast them for 30 seconds. Put the rest of the solid ingredients into the cup and press them down below the Max Line. Add the fluid base to fill the cup up to the Max Line. Screw the Nutribullet Extractor Blade on to the top of the cup. Invert the cup, press it down into the Nutribullet Power Base and twist it into place. Blast the mixture until it is really smooth (20 or so seconds). ***Enjoy!***

Lettuce and Orange Booster

Ingredients

1 Cup/Handful of Spinach (40 grams or 1½ oz)
1 Cup/Handful of Lettuce Leaves (40 grams or 1½ oz)
1 Cup of Orange segments (120 grams or 4 oz)
1 Cup of Strawberries (120 grams or 4 oz)
22 grams or ¾ oz of Flax Seeds
200 ml / 7 fl oz of Almond Milk (Unsweetened)

Protein 8g, Fat 12g, Carb 20g, Fibre 14g, 254 Kcals

Preparation

Place the nuts or seeds into the Tall Cup. Screw the Nutribullet Extractor Blade on to the top of the cup. Invert the cup, press it down into the Nutribullet Power Base and twist it into place. Blast them for 30 seconds. Put the rest of the solid ingredients into the cup and press them down below the Max Line. Add the fluid base to fill the cup up to the Max Line. Screw the Nutribullet Extractor Blade on to the top of the cup. Invert the cup, press it down into the Nutribullet Power Base and twist it into place. Blast the mixture until it is really smooth (20 or so seconds). ***Enjoy!***

Blueberry and Walnut Blend

Ingredients

1 Cup/Handful of Broccoli Florets (40 grams or 1½ oz)
1 Cup/Handful of Rocket/Arugura Lettuce (40 grams or 1½ oz)
1 Cup of Blueberries (120 grams or 4 oz)
1 Cup of Tangerine slices (120 grams or 4 oz)
30 grams or 1 oz of Walnuts
200 ml / 7 fl oz of Almond Milk (Unsweetened)

Protein 9g, Fat 23g, Carb 33g, Fibre 9g, 373 Kcals

Preparation

Place the nuts or seeds into the Tall Cup. Screw the Nutribullet Extractor Blade on to the top of the cup. Invert the cup, press it down into the Nutribullet Power Base and twist it into place. Blast them for 30 seconds. Put the rest of the solid ingredients into the cup and press them down below the Max Line. Add the fluid base to fill the cup up to the Max Line. Screw the Nutribullet Extractor Blade on to the top of the cup. Invert the cup, press it down into the Nutribullet Power Base and twist it into place. Blast the mixture until it is really smooth (20 or so seconds). **Enjoy!**

Lettuce and Sesame Medley

Ingredients

1 Cup/Handful of Spinach (40 grams or 1½ oz)
1 Cup/Handful of Lettuce Leaves (40 grams or 1½ oz)
1 Cup of Blackberries (120 grams or 4 oz)
1 Cup of Nectarine segments (120 grams or 4 oz)
22 grams or ¾ oz of Sesame Seeds Hulled
200 ml / 7 fl oz of Dairy Milk Semi Skimmed

Protein 16g, Fat 18g, Carb 27g, Fibre 12g, 351 Kcals

Preparation

Place the nuts or seeds into the Tall Cup. Screw the Nutribullet Extractor Blade on to the top of the cup. Invert the cup, press it down into the Nutribullet Power Base and twist it into place. Blast them for 30 seconds. Put the rest of the solid ingredients into the cup and press them down below the Max Line. Add the fluid base to fill the cup up to the Max Line. Screw the Nutribullet Extractor Blade on to the top of the cup. Invert the cup, press it down into the Nutribullet Power Base and twist it into place. Blast the mixture until it is really smooth (20 or so seconds). **Enjoy!**

Spinach befriends Blackberry

Ingredients

1 Cup/Handful of Spinach (40 grams or 1½ oz)
1 Cup/Handful of Lettuce Leaves (40 grams or 1½ oz)
1 Cup of Tangerine slices (120 grams or 4 oz)
1 Cup of Blackberries (120 grams or 4 oz)
22 grams or ¾ oz of Chia Seeds
200 ml / 7 fl oz of Dairy Milk Semi Skimmed

Protein 15g, Fat 12g, Carb 31g, Fibre 18g, 338 Kcals

Preparation

Place the nuts or seeds into the Tall Cup. Screw the Nutribullet Extractor Blade on to the top of the cup. Invert the cup, press it down into the Nutribullet Power Base and twist it into place. Blast them for 30 seconds. Put the rest of the solid ingredients into the cup and press them down below the Max Line. Add the fluid base to fill the cup up to the Max Line. Screw the Nutribullet Extractor Blade on to the top of the cup. Invert the cup, press it down into the Nutribullet Power Base and twist it into place. Blast the mixture until it is really smooth (20 or so seconds). **Enjoy!**

Orange and Pecan Salad

Ingredients

1 Cup/Handful of Broccoli Florets (40 grams or 1½ oz)
1 Cup/Handful of Rocket/Arugura Lettuce (40 grams or 1½ oz)
2 Cups of Orange segments (240 grams or 8 oz)
30 grams or 1 oz of Pecans
200 ml / 7 fl oz of Almond Milk (Unsweetened)

Protein 7g, Fat 24g, Carb 26g, Fibre 11g, 365 Kcals

Preparation

Place the nuts or seeds into the Tall Cup. Screw the Nutribullet Extractor Blade on to the top of the cup. Invert the cup, press it down into the Nutribullet Power Base and twist it into place. Blast them for 30 seconds. Put the rest of the solid ingredients into the cup and press them down below the Max Line. Add the fluid base to fill the cup up to the Max Line. Screw the Nutribullet Extractor Blade on to the top of the cup. Invert the cup, press it down into the Nutribullet Power Base and twist it into place. Blast the mixture until it is really smooth (20 or so seconds). **Enjoy!**

Raspberry Journey

Ingredients

1 Cup/Handful of Rocket/Arugura Lettuce (40 grams or 1½ oz)
1 Cup/Handful of Spinach (40 grams or 1½ oz)
1 Cup of Raspberries (120 grams or 4 oz)
1 Cup of Guava (120 grams or 4 oz)
22 grams or ¾ oz of Flax Seeds
200 ml / 7 fl oz of Dairy Milk Semi Skimmed

Protein 17g, Fat 15g, Carb 28g, Fibre 22g, 376 Kcals

Preparation

Place the nuts or seeds into the Tall Cup. Screw the Nutribullet Extractor Blade on to the top of the cup. Invert the cup, press it down into the Nutribullet Power Base and twist it into place. Blast them for 30 seconds. Put the rest of the solid ingredients into the cup and press them down below the Max Line. Add the fluid base to fill the cup up to the Max Line. Screw the Nutribullet Extractor Blade on to the top of the cup. Invert the cup, press it down into the Nutribullet Power Base and twist it into place. Blast the mixture until it is really smooth (20 or so seconds). **Enjoy!**

Nectarine Blossom

Ingredients

1 Cup/Handful of Broccoli Florets (40 grams or 1½ oz)
1 Cup/Handful of Lettuce Leaves (40 grams or 1½ oz)
1 Cup of Blueberries (120 grams or 4 oz)
1 Cup of Nectarine segments (120 grams or 4 oz)
30 grams or 1 oz of Walnuts
200 ml / 7 fl oz of Almond Milk (Unsweetened)

Protein 9g, Fat 23g, Carb 30g, Fibre 10g, 363 Kcals

Preparation

Place the nuts or seeds into the Tall Cup. Screw the Nutribullet Extractor Blade on to the top of the cup. Invert the cup, press it down into the Nutribullet Power Base and twist it into place. Blast them for 30 seconds. Put the rest of the solid ingredients into the cup and press them down below the Max Line. Add the fluid base to fill the cup up to the Max Line. Screw the Nutribullet Extractor Blade on to the top of the cup. Invert the cup, press it down into the Nutribullet Power Base and twist it into place. Blast the mixture until it is really smooth (20 or so seconds). **Enjoy!**

Strawberry and Sesame Melody

Ingredients

1 Cup/Handful of Rocket/Arugura Lettuce (40 grams or 1½ oz)
1 Cup/Handful of Broccoli Florets (40 grams or 1½ oz)
1 Cup of Strawberries (120 grams or 4 oz)
1 Cup of Orange segments (120 grams or 4 oz)
22 grams or ¾ oz of Sesame Seeds Hulled
200 ml / 7 fl oz of Almond Milk (Unsweetened)

Protein 8g, Fat 16g, Carb 21g, Fibre 9g, 271 Kcals

Preparation

Place the nuts or seeds into the Tall Cup. Screw the Nutribullet Extractor Blade on to the top of the cup. Invert the cup, press it down into the Nutribullet Power Base and twist it into place. Blast them for 30 seconds. Put the rest of the solid ingredients into the cup and press them down below the Max Line. Add the fluid base to fill the cup up to the Max Line. Screw the Nutribullet Extractor Blade on to the top of the cup. Invert the cup, press it down into the Nutribullet Power Base and twist it into place. Blast the mixture until it is really smooth (20 or so seconds). ***Enjoy!***

Strawberry and Chia Soother

Ingredients

1 Cup/Handful of Spinach (40 grams or 1½ oz)
1 Cup/Handful of Lettuce Leaves (40 grams or 1½ oz)
2 Cups of Strawberries (240 grams or 8 oz)
22 grams or ¾ oz of Chia Seeds
200 ml / 7 fl oz of Dairy Milk Semi Skimmed

Protein 14g, Fat 11g, Carb 26g, Fibre 14g, 299 Kcals

Preparation

Place the nuts or seeds into the Tall Cup. Screw the Nutribullet Extractor Blade on to the top of the cup. Invert the cup, press it down into the Nutribullet Power Base and twist it into place. Blast them for 30 seconds. Put the rest of the solid ingredients into the cup and press them down below the Max Line. Add the fluid base to fill the cup up to the Max Line. Screw the Nutribullet Extractor Blade on to the top of the cup. Invert the cup, press it down into the Nutribullet Power Base and twist it into place. Blast the mixture until it is really smooth (20 or so seconds). ***Enjoy!***

Tomato Vortex

Ingredients

2 Cups/Handfuls of Broccoli Florets (80 grams or 3 oz)
1 Cup of Strawberries (120 grams or 4 oz)
1 Cup of sliced Tomato (120 grams or 4 oz)
22 grams or ¾ oz of Flax Seeds
200 ml / 7 fl oz of Dairy Milk Semi Skimmed

Protein 15g, Fat 14g, Carb 23g, Fibre 12g, 304 Kcals

Preparation

Place the nuts or seeds into the Tall Cup. Screw the Nutribullet Extractor Blade on to the top of the cup. Invert the cup, press it down into the Nutribullet Power Base and twist it into place. Blast them for 30 seconds. Put the rest of the solid ingredients into the cup and press them down below the Max Line. Add the fluid base to fill the cup up to the Max Line. Screw the Nutribullet Extractor Blade on to the top of the cup. Invert the cup, press it down into the Nutribullet Power Base and twist it into place. Blast the mixture until it is really smooth (20 or so seconds). **Enjoy!**

Sesame Bonanza

Ingredients

2 Cups/Handfuls of Rocket/Arugura Lettuce (80 grams or 3 oz)
1 Cup of Guava (120 grams or 4 oz)
1 Cup of sliced Red Pepper (120 grams or 4 oz)
22 grams or ¾ oz of Sesame Seeds Hulled
200 ml / 7 fl oz of Almond Milk (Unsweetened)

Protein 10g, Fat 17g, Carb 17g, Fibre 13g, 288 Kcals

Preparation

Place the nuts or seeds into the Tall Cup. Screw the Nutribullet Extractor Blade on to the top of the cup. Invert the cup, press it down into the Nutribullet Power Base and twist it into place. Blast them for 30 seconds. Put the rest of the solid ingredients into the cup and press them down below the Max Line. Add the fluid base to fill the cup up to the Max Line. Screw the Nutribullet Extractor Blade on to the top of the cup. Invert the cup, press it down into the Nutribullet Power Base and twist it into place. Blast the mixture until it is really smooth (20 or so seconds). **Enjoy!**

Pecan Seduction

Ingredients

2 Cups/Handfuls of Lettuce Leaves (80 grams or 3 oz)
1 Cup of Orange segments (120 grams or 4 oz)
1 Cup of sliced Carrots (120 grams or 4 oz)
30 grams or 1 oz of Pecans
200 ml / 7 fl oz of Almond Milk (Unsweetened)

Protein 7g, Fat 24g, Carb 22g, Fibre 12g, 352 Kcals

Preparation

Place the nuts or seeds into the Tall Cup. Screw the Nutribullet Extractor Blade on to the top of the cup. Invert the cup, press it down into the Nutribullet Power Base and twist it into place. Blast them for 30 seconds. Put the rest of the solid ingredients into the cup and press them down below the Max Line. Add the fluid base to fill the cup up to the Max Line. Screw the Nutribullet Extractor Blade on to the top of the cup. Invert the cup, press it down into the Nutribullet Power Base and twist it into place. Blast the mixture until it is really smooth (20 or so seconds). **Enjoy!**

Nectarine and Cauliflower Delivered

Ingredients

2 Cups/Handfuls of Spinach (80 grams or 3 oz)
1 Cup of Nectarine segments (120 grams or 4 oz)
1 Cup of sliced Cauliflower florets (120 grams or 4 oz)
22 grams or ¾ oz of Chia Seeds
200 ml / 7 fl oz of Dairy Milk Semi Skimmed

Protein 17g, Fat 11g, Carb 27g, Fibre 14g, 308 Kcals

Preparation

Place the nuts or seeds into the Tall Cup. Screw the Nutribullet Extractor Blade on to the top of the cup. Invert the cup, press it down into the Nutribullet Power Base and twist it into place. Blast them for 30 seconds. Put the rest of the solid ingredients into the cup and press them down below the Max Line. Add the fluid base to fill the cup up to the Max Line. Screw the Nutribullet Extractor Blade on to the top of the cup. Invert the cup, press it down into the Nutribullet Power Base and twist it into place. Blast the mixture until it is really smooth (20 or so seconds). **Enjoy!**

Lettuce Fiesta

Ingredients

2 Cups/Handfuls of Lettuce Leaves (80 grams or 3 oz)
1 Cup of Blueberries (120 grams or 4 oz)
1 Cup of sliced Tomato (120 grams or 4 oz)
30 grams or 1 oz of Walnuts
200 ml / 7 fl oz of Dairy Milk Semi Skimmed

Protein 15g, Fat 24g, Carb 30g, Fibre 8g, 399 Kcals

Preparation

Place the nuts or seeds into the Tall Cup. Screw the Nutribullet Extractor Blade on to the top of the cup. Invert the cup, press it down into the Nutribullet Power Base and twist it into place. Blast them for 30 seconds. Put the rest of the solid ingredients into the cup and press them down below the Max Line. Add the fluid base to fill the cup up to the Max Line. Screw the Nutribullet Extractor Blade on to the top of the cup. Invert the cup, press it down into the Nutribullet Power Base and twist it into place. Blast the mixture until it is really smooth (20 or so seconds). **Enjoy!**

Red Pepper Paradise

Ingredients

1 Cup/Handful of Broccoli Florets (40 grams or 1½ oz)
1 Cup/Handful of Rocket/Arugura Lettuce (40 grams or 1½ oz)
1 Cup of Blackberries (120 grams or 4 oz)
1 Cup of sliced Red Pepper (120 grams or 4 oz)
30 grams or 1 oz of Pecans
200 ml / 7 fl oz of Almond Milk (Unsweetened)

Protein 8g, Fat 25g, Carb 14g, Fibre 14g, 341 Kcals

Preparation

Place the nuts or seeds into the Tall Cup. Screw the Nutribullet Extractor Blade on to the top of the cup. Invert the cup, press it down into the Nutribullet Power Base and twist it into place. Blast them for 30 seconds. Put the rest of the solid ingredients into the cup and press them down below the Max Line. Add the fluid base to fill the cup up to the Max Line. Screw the Nutribullet Extractor Blade on to the top of the cup. Invert the cup, press it down into the Nutribullet Power Base and twist it into place. Blast the mixture until it is really smooth (20 or so seconds). **Enjoy!**

Raspberry meets Cauliflower

Ingredients

2 Cups/Handfuls of Spinach (80 grams or 3 oz)
1 Cup of Raspberries (120 grams or 4 oz)
1 Cup of sliced Cauliflower florets (120 grams or 4 oz)
22 grams or ¾ oz of Flax Seeds
200 ml / 7 fl oz of Dairy Milk Semi Skimmed

Protein 17g, Fat 14g, Carb 21g, Fibre 18g, 328 Kcals

Preparation

Place the nuts or seeds into the Tall Cup. Screw the Nutribullet Extractor Blade on to the top of the cup. Invert the cup, press it down into the Nutribullet Power Base and twist it into place. Blast them for 30 seconds. Put the rest of the solid ingredients into the cup and press them down below the Max Line. Add the fluid base to fill the cup up to the Max Line. Screw the Nutribullet Extractor Blade on to the top of the cup. Invert the cup, press it down into the Nutribullet Power Base and twist it into place. Blast the mixture until it is really smooth (20 or so seconds). *Enjoy!*

Spinach Orchard

Ingredients

1 Cup/Handful of Lettuce Leaves (40 grams or 1½ oz)
1 Cup/Handful of Spinach (40 grams or 1½ oz)
1 Cup of Tangerine slices (120 grams or 4 oz)
1 Cup of sliced Carrots (120 grams or 4 oz)
30 grams or 1 oz of Walnuts
200 ml / 7 fl oz of Almond Milk (Unsweetened)

Protein 9g, Fat 23g, Carb 25g, Fibre 10g, 350 Kcals

Preparation

Place the nuts or seeds into the Tall Cup. Screw the Nutribullet Extractor Blade on to the top of the cup. Invert the cup, press it down into the Nutribullet Power Base and twist it into place. Blast them for 30 seconds. Put the rest of the solid ingredients into the cup and press them down below the Max Line. Add the fluid base to fill the cup up to the Max Line. Screw the Nutribullet Extractor Blade on to the top of the cup. Invert the cup, press it down into the Nutribullet Power Base and twist it into place. Blast the mixture until it is really smooth (20 or so seconds). *Enjoy!*

Broccoli befriends Chia

Ingredients

1 Cup/Handful of Broccoli Florets (40 grams or 1½ oz)
1 Cup/Handful of Spinach (40 grams or 1½ oz)
1 Cup of Guava (120 grams or 4 oz)
1 Cup of sliced Carrots (120 grams or 4 oz)
22 grams or ¾ oz of Chia Seeds
200 ml / 7 fl oz of Almond Milk (Unsweetened)

Protein 11g, Fat 11g, Carb 23g, Fibre 20g, 286 Kcals

Preparation

Place the nuts or seeds into the Tall Cup. Screw the Nutribullet Extractor Blade on to the top of the cup. Invert the cup, press it down into the Nutribullet Power Base and twist it into place. Blast them for 30 seconds. Put the rest of the solid ingredients into the cup and press them down below the Max Line. Add the fluid base to fill the cup up to the Max Line. Screw the Nutribullet Extractor Blade on to the top of the cup. Invert the cup, press it down into the Nutribullet Power Base and twist it into place. Blast the mixture until it is really smooth (20 or so seconds). **Enjoy!**

Raspberry Heaven

Ingredients

1 Cup/Handful of Rocket/Arugura Lettuce (40 grams or 1½ oz)
1 Cup/Handful of Lettuce Leaves (40 grams or 1½ oz)
1 Cup of Raspberries (120 grams or 4 oz)
1 Cup of sliced Red Pepper (120 grams or 4 oz)
22 grams or ¾ oz of Sesame Seeds Hulled
200 ml / 7 fl oz of Dairy Milk Semi Skimmed

Protein 15g, Fat 18g, Carb 22g, Fibre 13g, 343 Kcals

Preparation

Place the nuts or seeds into the Tall Cup. Screw the Nutribullet Extractor Blade on to the top of the cup. Invert the cup, press it down into the Nutribullet Power Base and twist it into place. Blast them for 30 seconds. Put the rest of the solid ingredients into the cup and press them down below the Max Line. Add the fluid base to fill the cup up to the Max Line. Screw the Nutribullet Extractor Blade on to the top of the cup. Invert the cup, press it down into the Nutribullet Power Base and twist it into place. Blast the mixture until it is really smooth (20 or so seconds). **Enjoy!**

Blasts for Deeper Longer Sleep and Happiness
High in Tryptophan, Magnesium, Vitamins B3, B6, B9

Beetroot Sensation

Ingredients

1 Cup/Handful of Spinach (40 grams or 1½ oz)
1 Cup/Handful of Broccoli Florets (40 grams or 1½ oz)
1 Cup of Apricot halves (120 grams or 4 oz)
1 Cup of diced Beetroot (120 grams or 4 oz)
30 grams or 1 oz of Walnuts
200 ml / 7 fl oz of Dairy Milk Semi Skimmed

Protein 18g, Fat 24g, Carb 33g, Fibre 10g, 428 Kcals

Preparation

Place the nuts or seeds into the Tall Cup. Screw the Nutribullet Extractor Blade on to the top of the cup. Invert the cup, press it down into the Nutribullet Power Base and twist it into place. Blast them for 30 seconds. Put the rest of the solid ingredients into the cup and press them down below the Max Line. Add the fluid base to fill the cup up to the Max Line. Screw the Nutribullet Extractor Blade on to the top of the cup. Invert the cup, press it down into the Nutribullet Power Base and twist it into place. Blast the mixture until it is really smooth (20 or so seconds). *Enjoy!*

Prune kisses Pumpkin

Ingredients

1 Cup/Handful of Watercress (40 grams or 1½ oz)
1 Cup/Handful of Spinach (40 grams or 1½ oz)
1 Cup of Prunes (stoned) (120 grams or 4 oz)
1 Cup of sliced Carrots (120 grams or 4 oz)
22 grams or ¾ oz of Pumpkin Seeds
200 ml / 7 fl oz of Almond Milk (Unsweetened)

Protein 10g, Fat 14g, Carb 15g, Fibre 9g, 218 Kcals

Preparation

Place the nuts or seeds into the Tall Cup. Screw the Nutribullet Extractor Blade on to the top of the cup. Invert the cup, press it down into the Nutribullet Power Base and twist it into place. Blast them for 30 seconds. Put the rest of the solid ingredients into the cup and press them down below the Max Line. Add the fluid base to fill the cup up to the Max Line. Screw the Nutribullet Extractor Blade on to the top of the cup. Invert the cup, press it down into the Nutribullet Power Base and twist it into place. Blast the mixture until it is really smooth (20 or so seconds). *Enjoy!*

Watercress Fiesta

Ingredients

1 Cup/Handful of Watercress (40 grams or 1½ oz)
1 Cup/Handful of Broccoli Florets (40 grams or 1½ oz)
1 small Avocado (stoned and peeled) (120 grams or 4 oz)
1 Cup of sliced Fine Beans (120 grams or 4 oz)
22 grams or ¾ oz of Chia Seeds
200 ml / 7 fl oz of Dairy Milk Semi Skimmed

Protein 18g, Fat 29g, Carb 19g, Fibre 19g, 446 Kcals

Preparation

Place the nuts or seeds into the Tall Cup. Screw the Nutribullet Extractor Blade on to the top of the cup. Invert the cup, press it down into the Nutribullet Power Base and twist it into place. Blast them for 30 seconds. Put the rest of the solid ingredients into the cup and press them down below the Max Line. Add the fluid base to fill the cup up to the Max Line. Screw the Nutribullet Extractor Blade on to the top of the cup. Invert the cup, press it down into the Nutribullet Power Base and twist it into place. Blast the mixture until it is really smooth (20 or so seconds). *Enjoy!*

Apricot befriends Sunflower

Ingredients

1 Cup/Handful of Watercress (40 grams or 1½ oz)
1 Cup/Handful of Broccoli Florets (40 grams or 1½ oz)
1 Cup of Apricot halves (120 grams or 4 oz)
1 Cup of sliced Cauliflower florets (120 grams or 4 oz)
22 grams or ¾ oz of Sunflower Seeds Hulled
200 ml / 7 fl oz of Almond Milk (Unsweetened)

Protein 11g, Fat 14g, Carb 19g, Fibre 8g, 245 Kcals

Preparation

Place the nuts or seeds into the Tall Cup. Screw the Nutribullet Extractor Blade on to the top of the cup. Invert the cup, press it down into the Nutribullet Power Base and twist it into place. Blast them for 30 seconds. Put the rest of the solid ingredients into the cup and press them down below the Max Line. Add the fluid base to fill the cup up to the Max Line. Screw the Nutribullet Extractor Blade on to the top of the cup. Invert the cup, press it down into the Nutribullet Power Base and twist it into place. Blast the mixture until it is really smooth (20 or so seconds). *Enjoy!*

Prune and Beetroot Sunrise

Ingredients

1 Cup/Handful of Spinach (40 grams or 1½ oz)
1 Cup/Handful of Broccoli Florets (40 grams or 1½ oz)
1 Cup of Prunes (stoned) (120 grams or 4 oz)
1 Cup of diced Beetroot (120 grams or 4 oz)
22 grams or ¾ oz of Sesame Seeds Hulled
200 ml / 7 fl oz of Almond Milk (Unsweetened)

Protein 10g, Fat 17g, Carb 15g, Fibre 11g, 236 Kcals

Preparation

Place the nuts or seeds into the Tall Cup. Screw the Nutribullet Extractor Blade on to the top of the cup. Invert the cup, press it down into the Nutribullet Power Base and twist it into place. Blast them for 30 seconds. Put the rest of the solid ingredients into the cup and press them down below the Max Line. Add the fluid base to fill the cup up to the Max Line. Screw the Nutribullet Extractor Blade on to the top of the cup. Invert the cup, press it down into the Nutribullet Power Base and twist it into place. Blast the mixture until it is really smooth (20 or so seconds). **Enjoy!**

Spinach Royale

Ingredients

1 Cup/Handful of Spinach (40 grams or 1½ oz)
1 Cup/Handful of Watercress (40 grams or 1½ oz)
1 small Avocado (stoned and peeled) (120 grams or 4 oz)
1 Cup of sliced Fine Beans (120 grams or 4 oz)
30 grams or 1 oz of Cashews
200 ml / 7 fl oz of Dairy Milk Semi Skimmed

Protein 19g, Fat 35g, Carb 25g, Fibre 13g, 501 Kcals

Preparation

Place the nuts or seeds into the Tall Cup. Screw the Nutribullet Extractor Blade on to the top of the cup. Invert the cup, press it down into the Nutribullet Power Base and twist it into place. Blast them for 30 seconds. Put the rest of the solid ingredients into the cup and press them down below the Max Line. Add the fluid base to fill the cup up to the Max Line. Screw the Nutribullet Extractor Blade on to the top of the cup. Invert the cup, press it down into the Nutribullet Power Base and twist it into place. Blast the mixture until it is really smooth (20 or so seconds). **Enjoy!**

Watercress and Apricot Tango

Ingredients

2 Cups/Handfuls of Watercress (80 grams or 3 oz)
1 Cup of Apricot halves (120 grams or 4 oz)
1 Cup of sliced Cauliflower florets (120 grams or 4 oz)
30 grams or 1 oz of Peanuts
200 ml / 7 fl oz of Almond Milk (Unsweetened)

Protein 14g, Fat 18g, Carb 18g, Fibre 9g, 292 Kcals

Preparation

Place the nuts or seeds into the Tall Cup. Screw the Nutribullet Extractor Blade on to the top of the cup. Invert the cup, press it down into the Nutribullet Power Base and twist it into place. Blast them for 30 seconds. Put the rest of the solid ingredients into the cup and press them down below the Max Line. Add the fluid base to fill the cup up to the Max Line. Screw the Nutribullet Extractor Blade on to the top of the cup. Invert the cup, press it down into the Nutribullet Power Base and twist it into place. Blast the mixture until it is really smooth (20 or so seconds). **Enjoy!**

Prune embraces Carrot

Ingredients

1 Cup/Handful of Spinach (40 grams or 1½ oz)
1 Cup/Handful of Broccoli Florets (40 grams or 1½ oz)
1 Cup of Prunes (stoned) (120 grams or 4 oz)
1 Cup of sliced Carrots (120 grams or 4 oz)
30 grams or 1 oz of Peanuts
200 ml / 7 fl oz of Dairy Milk Semi Skimmed

Protein 19g, Fat 21g, Carb 26g, Fibre 11g, 347 Kcals

Preparation

Place the nuts or seeds into the Tall Cup. Screw the Nutribullet Extractor Blade on to the top of the cup. Invert the cup, press it down into the Nutribullet Power Base and twist it into place. Blast them for 30 seconds. Put the rest of the solid ingredients into the cup and press them down below the Max Line. Add the fluid base to fill the cup up to the Max Line. Screw the Nutribullet Extractor Blade on to the top of the cup. Invert the cup, press it down into the Nutribullet Power Base and twist it into place. Blast the mixture until it is really smooth (20 or so seconds). **Enjoy!**

Broccoli Morning

Ingredients

1 Cup/Handful of Watercress (40 grams or 1½ oz)
1 Cup/Handful of Broccoli Florets (40 grams or 1½ oz)
1 small Avocado (stoned and peeled) (120 grams or 4 oz)
1 Cup of sliced Carrots (120 grams or 4 oz)
30 grams or 1 oz of Walnuts
200 ml / 7 fl oz of Almond Milk (Unsweetened)

Protein 11g, Fat 40g, Carb 15g, Fibre 15g, 481 Kcals

Preparation

Place the nuts or seeds into the Tall Cup. Screw the Nutribullet Extractor Blade on to the top of the cup. Invert the cup, press it down into the Nutribullet Power Base and twist it into place. Blast them for 30 seconds. Put the rest of the solid ingredients into the cup and press them down below the Max Line. Add the fluid base to fill the cup up to the Max Line. Screw the Nutribullet Extractor Blade on to the top of the cup. Invert the cup, press it down into the Nutribullet Power Base and twist it into place. Blast the mixture until it is really smooth (20 or so seconds). **Enjoy!**

Spinach invites Watercress

Ingredients

1 Cup/Handful of Spinach (40 grams or 1½ oz)
1 Cup/Handful of Watercress (40 grams or 1½ oz)
1 Cup of Apricot halves (120 grams or 4 oz)
1 Cup of diced Beetroot (120 grams or 4 oz)
22 grams or ¾ oz of Sunflower Seeds Hulled
200 ml / 7 fl oz of Dairy Milk Semi Skimmed

Protein 17g, Fat 15g, Carb 32g, Fibre 8g, 336 Kcals

Preparation

Place the nuts or seeds into the Tall Cup. Screw the Nutribullet Extractor Blade on to the top of the cup. Invert the cup, press it down into the Nutribullet Power Base and twist it into place. Blast them for 30 seconds. Put the rest of the solid ingredients into the cup and press them down below the Max Line. Add the fluid base to fill the cup up to the Max Line. Screw the Nutribullet Extractor Blade on to the top of the cup. Invert the cup, press it down into the Nutribullet Power Base and twist it into place. Blast the mixture until it is really smooth (20 or so seconds). **Enjoy!**

Fine Bean Dance

Ingredients

2 Cups/Handfuls of Broccoli Florets (80 grams or 3 oz)
1 small Avocado (stoned and peeled) (120 grams or 4 oz)
1 Cup of sliced Fine Beans (120 grams or 4 oz)
22 grams or ¾ oz of Chia Seeds
200 ml / 7 fl oz of Almond Milk (Unsweetened)

Protein 11g, Fat 27g, Carb 11g, Fibre 21g, 382 Kcals

Preparation

Place the nuts or seeds into the Tall Cup. Screw the Nutribullet Extractor Blade on to the top of the cup. Invert the cup, press it down into the Nutribullet Power Base and twist it into place. Blast them for 30 seconds. Put the rest of the solid ingredients into the cup and press them down below the Max Line. Add the fluid base to fill the cup up to the Max Line. Screw the Nutribullet Extractor Blade on to the top of the cup. Invert the cup, press it down into the Nutribullet Power Base and twist it into place. Blast the mixture until it is really smooth (20 or so seconds). **Enjoy!**

Pumpkin Delusion

Ingredients

2 Cups/Handfuls of Watercress (80 grams or 3 oz)
1 Cup of Prunes (stoned) (120 grams or 4 oz)
1 Cup of sliced Cauliflower florets (120 grams or 4 oz)
22 grams or ¾ oz of Pumpkin Seeds
200 ml / 7 fl oz of Dairy Milk Semi Skimmed

Protein 18g, Fat 16g, Carb 20g, Fibre 7g, 268 Kcals

Preparation

Place the nuts or seeds into the Tall Cup. Screw the Nutribullet Extractor Blade on to the top of the cup. Invert the cup, press it down into the Nutribullet Power Base and twist it into place. Blast them for 30 seconds. Put the rest of the solid ingredients into the cup and press them down below the Max Line. Add the fluid base to fill the cup up to the Max Line. Screw the Nutribullet Extractor Blade on to the top of the cup. Invert the cup, press it down into the Nutribullet Power Base and twist it into place. Blast the mixture until it is really smooth (20 or so seconds). **Enjoy!**

Avocado in Cashew

Ingredients

1 Cup/Handful of Watercress (40 grams or 1½ oz)
1 Cup/Handful of Spinach (40 grams or 1½ oz)
1 small Avocado (stoned and peeled) (120 grams or 4 oz)
1 Cup of sliced Cauliflower florets (120 grams or 4 oz)
30 grams or 1 oz of Cashews
200 ml / 7 fl oz of Dairy Milk Semi Skimmed

Protein 19g, Fat 35g, Carb 24g, Fibre 13g, 501 Kcals

Preparation

Place the nuts or seeds into the Tall Cup. Screw the Nutribullet Extractor Blade on to the top of the cup. Invert the cup, press it down into the Nutribullet Power Base and twist it into place. Blast them for 30 seconds. Put the rest of the solid ingredients into the cup and press them down below the Max Line. Add the fluid base to fill the cup up to the Max Line. Screw the Nutribullet Extractor Blade on to the top of the cup. Invert the cup, press it down into the Nutribullet Power Base and twist it into place. Blast the mixture until it is really smooth (20 or so seconds). **Enjoy!**

Prune Embrace

Ingredients

1 Cup/Handful of Broccoli Florets (40 grams or 1½ oz)
1 Cup/Handful of Watercress (40 grams or 1½ oz)
1 Cup of Prunes (stoned) (120 grams or 4 oz)
1 Cup of sliced Carrots (120 grams or 4 oz)
22 grams or ¾ oz of Sesame Seeds Hulled
200 ml / 7 fl oz of Almond Milk (Unsweetened)

Protein 9g, Fat 17g, Carb 14g, Fibre 10g, 229 Kcals

Preparation

Place the nuts or seeds into the Tall Cup. Screw the Nutribullet Extractor Blade on to the top of the cup. Invert the cup, press it down into the Nutribullet Power Base and twist it into place. Blast them for 30 seconds. Put the rest of the solid ingredients into the cup and press them down below the Max Line. Add the fluid base to fill the cup up to the Max Line. Screw the Nutribullet Extractor Blade on to the top of the cup. Invert the cup, press it down into the Nutribullet Power Base and twist it into place. Blast the mixture until it is really smooth (20 or so seconds). **Enjoy!**

Apricot Blend

Ingredients

1 Cup/Handful of Broccoli Florets (40 grams or 1½ oz)
1 Cup/Handful of Watercress (40 grams or 1½ oz)
1 Cup of Apricot halves (120 grams or 4 oz)
1 Cup of sliced Fine Beans (120 grams or 4 oz)
22 grams or ¾ oz of Sunflower Seeds Hulled
200 ml / 7 fl oz of Almond Milk (Unsweetened)

Protein 11g, Fat 14g, Carb 20g, Fibre 8g, 245 Kcals

Preparation

Place the nuts or seeds into the Tall Cup. Screw the Nutribullet Extractor Blade on to the top of the cup. Invert the cup, press it down into the Nutribullet Power Base and twist it into place. Blast them for 30 seconds. Put the rest of the solid ingredients into the cup and press them down below the Max Line. Add the fluid base to fill the cup up to the Max Line. Screw the Nutribullet Extractor Blade on to the top of the cup. Invert the cup, press it down into the Nutribullet Power Base and twist it into place. Blast the mixture until it is really smooth (20 or so seconds). **Enjoy!**

Watercress and Broccoli Constellation

Ingredients

1 Cup/Handful of Watercress (40 grams or 1½ oz)
1 Cup/Handful of Broccoli Florets (40 grams or 1½ oz)
1 small Avocado (stoned and peeled) (120 grams or 4 oz)
1 Cup of sliced Cauliflower florets (120 grams or 4 oz)
22 grams or ¾ oz of Pumpkin Seeds
200 ml / 7 fl oz of Dairy Milk Semi Skimmed

Protein 19g, Fat 31g, Carb 19g, Fibre 13g, 464 Kcals

Preparation

Place the nuts or seeds into the Tall Cup. Screw the Nutribullet Extractor Blade on to the top of the cup. Invert the cup, press it down into the Nutribullet Power Base and twist it into place. Blast them for 30 seconds. Put the rest of the solid ingredients into the cup and press them down below the Max Line. Add the fluid base to fill the cup up to the Max Line. Screw the Nutribullet Extractor Blade on to the top of the cup. Invert the cup, press it down into the Nutribullet Power Base and twist it into place. Blast the mixture until it is really smooth (20 or so seconds). **Enjoy!**

Carrot Consortium

Ingredients

2 Cups/Handfuls of Spinach (80 grams or 3 oz)
1 Cup of Prunes (stoned) (120 grams or 4 oz)
1 Cup of sliced Carrots (120 grams or 4 oz)
22 grams or ¾ oz of Sesame Seeds Hulled
200 ml / 7 fl oz of Dairy Milk Semi Skimmed

Protein 16g, Fat 19g, Carb 23g, Fibre 10g, 304 Kcals

Preparation

Place the nuts or seeds into the Tall Cup. Screw the Nutribullet Extractor Blade on to the top of the cup. Invert the cup, press it down into the Nutribullet Power Base and twist it into place. Blast them for 30 seconds. Put the rest of the solid ingredients into the cup and press them down below the Max Line. Add the fluid base to fill the cup up to the Max Line. Screw the Nutribullet Extractor Blade on to the top of the cup. Invert the cup, press it down into the Nutribullet Power Base and twist it into place. Blast the mixture until it is really smooth (20 or so seconds). **Enjoy!**

Broccoli meets Prune

Ingredients

1 Cup/Handful of Spinach (40 grams or 1½ oz)
1 Cup/Handful of Broccoli Florets (40 grams or 1½ oz)
1 Cup of Prunes (stoned) (120 grams or 4 oz)
1 Cup of sliced Fine Beans (120 grams or 4 oz)
22 grams or ¾ oz of Sunflower Seeds Hulled
200 ml / 7 fl oz of Almond Milk (Unsweetened)

Protein 11g, Fat 16g, Carb 13g, Fibre 10g, 197 Kcals

Preparation

Place the nuts or seeds into the Tall Cup. Screw the Nutribullet Extractor Blade on to the top of the cup. Invert the cup, press it down into the Nutribullet Power Base and twist it into place. Blast them for 30 seconds. Put the rest of the solid ingredients into the cup and press them down below the Max Line. Add the fluid base to fill the cup up to the Max Line. Screw the Nutribullet Extractor Blade on to the top of the cup. Invert the cup, press it down into the Nutribullet Power Base and twist it into place. Blast the mixture until it is really smooth (20 or so seconds). **Enjoy!**

Sesame Mirage

Ingredients

1 Cup/Handful of Watercress (40 grams or 1½ oz)
1 Cup/Handful of Broccoli Florets (40 grams or 1½ oz)
1 Cup of Prunes (stoned) (120 grams or 4 oz)
1 Cup of sliced Fine Beans (120 grams or 4 oz)
22 grams or ¾ oz of Sesame Seeds Hulled
200 ml / 7 fl oz of Almond Milk (Unsweetened)

Protein 10g, Fat 18g, Carb 10g, Fibre 9g, 210 Kcals

Preparation

Place the nuts or seeds into the Tall Cup. Screw the Nutribullet Extractor Blade on to the top of the cup. Invert the cup, press it down into the Nutribullet Power Base and twist it into place. Blast them for 30 seconds. Put the rest of the solid ingredients into the cup and press them down below the Max Line. Add the fluid base to fill the cup up to the Max Line. Screw the Nutribullet Extractor Blade on to the top of the cup. Invert the cup, press it down into the Nutribullet Power Base and twist it into place. Blast the mixture until it is really smooth (20 or so seconds). **Enjoy!**

Apricot and Cashew Contradiction

Ingredients

1 Cup/Handful of Broccoli Florets (40 grams or 1½ oz)
1 Cup/Handful of Spinach (40 grams or 1½ oz)
1 Cup of Apricot halves (120 grams or 4 oz)
1 Cup of sliced Carrots (120 grams or 4 oz)
30 grams or 1 oz of Cashews
200 ml / 7 fl oz of Dairy Milk Semi Skimmed

Protein 18g, Fat 18g, Carb 39g, Fibre 9g, 395 Kcals

Preparation

Place the nuts or seeds into the Tall Cup. Screw the Nutribullet Extractor Blade on to the top of the cup. Invert the cup, press it down into the Nutribullet Power Base and twist it into place. Blast them for 30 seconds. Put the rest of the solid ingredients into the cup and press them down below the Max Line. Add the fluid base to fill the cup up to the Max Line. Screw the Nutribullet Extractor Blade on to the top of the cup. Invert the cup, press it down into the Nutribullet Power Base and twist it into place. Blast the mixture until it is really smooth (20 or so seconds). **Enjoy!**

Strawberry goes Walnut

Ingredients

2 Cups/Handfuls of Green Cabbage (80 grams or 3 oz)
1 Cup of Blueberries (120 grams or 4 oz)
1 Cup of Strawberries (120 grams or 4 oz)
30 grams or 1 oz of Walnuts
200 ml / 7 fl oz of Hazelnut Milk

Protein 8g, Fat 24g, Carb 32g, Fibre 10g, 380 Kcals

Preparation

Place the nuts or seeds into the Tall Cup. Screw the Nutribullet Extractor Blade on to the top of the cup. Invert the cup, press it down into the Nutribullet Power Base and twist it into place. Blast them for 30 seconds. Put the rest of the solid ingredients into the cup and press them down below the Max Line. Add the fluid base to fill the cup up to the Max Line. Screw the Nutribullet Extractor Blade on to the top of the cup. Invert the cup, press it down into the Nutribullet Power Base and twist it into place. Blast the mixture until it is really smooth (20 or so seconds). ***Enjoy!***

Rocket partners Pumpkin

Ingredients

2 Cups/Handfuls of Rocket/Arugura Lettuce (80 grams or 3 oz)
1 small Avocado (stoned and peeled) (120 grams or 4 oz)
1 Cup of Blackberries (120 grams or 4 oz)
22 grams or ¾ oz of Pumpkin Seeds
200 ml / 7 fl oz of Almond Milk (Unsweetened)

Protein 11g, Fat 30g, Carb 11g, Fibre 17g, 405 Kcals

Preparation

Place the nuts or seeds into the Tall Cup. Screw the Nutribullet Extractor Blade on to the top of the cup. Invert the cup, press it down into the Nutribullet Power Base and twist it into place. Blast them for 30 seconds. Put the rest of the solid ingredients into the cup and press them down below the Max Line. Add the fluid base to fill the cup up to the Max Line. Screw the Nutribullet Extractor Blade on to the top of the cup. Invert the cup, press it down into the Nutribullet Power Base and twist it into place. Blast the mixture until it is really smooth (20 or so seconds). ***Enjoy!***

Blueberry and Brazil Morning

Ingredients

1 Cup/Handful of Bok Choy (40 grams or 1½ oz)
1 Cup/Handful of Green Cabbage (40 grams or 1½ oz)
1 Cup of Blueberries (120 grams or 4 oz)
1 Cup of Strawberries (120 grams or 4 oz)
30 grams or 1 oz of Brazil nuts
200 ml / 7 fl oz of Water

Protein 7g, Fat 21g, Carb 24g, Fibre 9g, 319 Kcals

Preparation

Place the nuts or seeds into the Tall Cup. Screw the Nutribullet Extractor Blade on to the top of the cup. Invert the cup, press it down into the Nutribullet Power Base and twist it into place. Blast them for 30 seconds. Put the rest of the solid ingredients into the cup and press them down below the Max Line. Add the fluid base to fill the cup up to the Max Line. Screw the Nutribullet Extractor Blade on to the top of the cup. Invert the cup, press it down into the Nutribullet Power Base and twist it into place. Blast the mixture until it is really smooth (20 or so seconds). *Enjoy!*

Blackberry Booster

Ingredients

1 Cup/Handful of Spinach (40 grams or 1½ oz)
1 Cup/Handful of Mint (40 grams or 1½ oz)
1 Cup of Blackberries (120 grams or 4 oz)
1 small Avocado (stoned and peeled) (120 grams or 4 oz)
30 grams or 1 oz of Pecans
200 ml / 7 fl oz of Coconut Milk

Protein 9g, Fat 42g, Carb 15g, Fibre 21g, 517 Kcals

Preparation

Place the nuts or seeds into the Tall Cup. Screw the Nutribullet Extractor Blade on to the top of the cup. Invert the cup, press it down into the Nutribullet Power Base and twist it into place. Blast them for 30 seconds. Put the rest of the solid ingredients into the cup and press them down below the Max Line. Add the fluid base to fill the cup up to the Max Line. Screw the Nutribullet Extractor Blade on to the top of the cup. Invert the cup, press it down into the Nutribullet Power Base and twist it into place. Blast the mixture until it is really smooth (20 or so seconds). *Enjoy!*

Rocket and Strawberry Fandango

Ingredients

1 Cup/Handful of Rocket/Arugura Lettuce (40 grams or 1½ oz)
1 Cup/Handful of Watercress (40 grams or 1½ oz)
2 Cups of Strawberries (240 grams or 8 oz)
22 grams or ¾ oz of Flax Seeds
200 ml / 7 fl oz of Hazelnut Milk

Protein 8g, Fat 13g, Carb 21g, Fibre 12g, 262 Kcals

Preparation

Place the nuts or seeds into the Tall Cup. Screw the Nutribullet Extractor Blade on to the top of the cup. Invert the cup, press it down into the Nutribullet Power Base and twist it into place. Blast them for 30 seconds. Put the rest of the solid ingredients into the cup and press them down below the Max Line. Add the fluid base to fill the cup up to the Max Line. Screw the Nutribullet Extractor Blade on to the top of the cup. Invert the cup, press it down into the Nutribullet Power Base and twist it into place. Blast the mixture until it is really smooth (20 or so seconds). **Enjoy!**

Bok Choy and Avocado Melody

Ingredients

1 Cup/Handful of Bok Choy (40 grams or 1½ oz)
1 Cup/Handful of Watercress (40 grams or 1½ oz)
1 small Avocado (stoned and peeled) (120 grams or 4 oz)
1 Cup of Blackberries (120 grams or 4 oz)
30 grams or 1 oz of Cashews
200 ml / 7 fl oz of Almond Milk (Unsweetened)

Protein 12g, Fat 34g, Carb 16g, Fibre 17g, 445 Kcals

Preparation

Place the nuts or seeds into the Tall Cup. Screw the Nutribullet Extractor Blade on to the top of the cup. Invert the cup, press it down into the Nutribullet Power Base and twist it into place. Blast them for 30 seconds. Put the rest of the solid ingredients into the cup and press them down below the Max Line. Add the fluid base to fill the cup up to the Max Line. Screw the Nutribullet Extractor Blade on to the top of the cup. Invert the cup, press it down into the Nutribullet Power Base and twist it into place. Blast the mixture until it is really smooth (20 or so seconds). **Enjoy!**

Hazelnut Debut

Ingredients

1 Cup/Handful of Green Cabbage (40 grams or 1½ oz)
1 Cup/Handful of Mint (40 grams or 1½ oz)
1 Cup of Strawberries (120 grams or 4 oz)
1 Cup of Blueberries (120 grams or 4 oz)
30 grams or 1 oz of Hazelnuts
200 ml / 7 fl oz of Water

Protein 8g, Fat 19g, Carb 25g, Fibre 12g, 322 Kcals

Preparation

Place the nuts or seeds into the Tall Cup. Screw the Nutribullet Extractor Blade on to the top of the cup. Invert the cup, press it down into the Nutribullet Power Base and twist it into place. Blast them for 30 seconds. Put the rest of the solid ingredients into the cup and press them down below the Max Line. Add the fluid base to fill the cup up to the Max Line. Screw the Nutribullet Extractor Blade on to the top of the cup. Invert the cup, press it down into the Nutribullet Power Base and twist it into place. Blast the mixture until it is really smooth (20 or so seconds). **Enjoy!**

Green Cabbage Delight

Ingredients

2 Cups/Handfuls of Green Cabbage (80 grams or 3 oz)
1 Cup of Strawberries (120 grams or 4 oz)
1 Cup of Blackberries (120 grams or 4 oz)
30 grams or 1 oz of Almonds
200 ml / 7 fl oz of Coconut Milk

Protein 10g, Fat 19g, Carb 22g, Fibre 14g, 327 Kcals

Preparation

Place the nuts or seeds into the Tall Cup. Screw the Nutribullet Extractor Blade on to the top of the cup. Invert the cup, press it down into the Nutribullet Power Base and twist it into place. Blast them for 30 seconds. Put the rest of the solid ingredients into the cup and press them down below the Max Line. Add the fluid base to fill the cup up to the Max Line. Screw the Nutribullet Extractor Blade on to the top of the cup. Invert the cup, press it down into the Nutribullet Power Base and twist it into place. Blast the mixture until it is really smooth (20 or so seconds). **Enjoy!**

Rocket and Blueberry Journey

Ingredients

1 Cup/Handful of Spinach (40 grams or 1½ oz)
1 Cup/Handful of Rocket/Arugura Lettuce (40 grams or 1½ oz)
1 small Avocado (stoned and peeled) (120 grams or 4 oz)
1 Cup of Blueberries (120 grams or 4 oz)
22 grams or ¾ oz of Sesame Seeds Hulled
200 ml / 7 fl oz of Hazelnut Milk

Protein 10g, Fat 34g, Carb 24g, Fibre 15g, 465 Kcals

Preparation

Place the nuts or seeds into the Tall Cup. Screw the Nutribullet Extractor Blade on to the top of the cup. Invert the cup, press it down into the Nutribullet Power Base and twist it into place. Blast them for 30 seconds. Put the rest of the solid ingredients into the cup and press them down below the Max Line. Add the fluid base to fill the cup up to the Max Line. Screw the Nutribullet Extractor Blade on to the top of the cup. Invert the cup, press it down into the Nutribullet Power Base and twist it into place. Blast the mixture until it is really smooth (20 or so seconds). **Enjoy!**

Blueberry and Almond Royale

Ingredients

2 Cups/Handfuls of Bok Choy (80 grams or 3 oz)
1 small Avocado (stoned and peeled) (120 grams or 4 oz)
1 Cup of Blueberries (120 grams or 4 oz)
30 grams or 1 oz of Almonds
200 ml / 7 fl oz of Almond Milk (Unsweetened)

Protein 12g, Fat 36g, Carb 20g, Fibre 16g, 473 Kcals

Preparation

Place the nuts or seeds into the Tall Cup. Screw the Nutribullet Extractor Blade on to the top of the cup. Invert the cup, press it down into the Nutribullet Power Base and twist it into place. Blast them for 30 seconds. Put the rest of the solid ingredients into the cup and press them down below the Max Line. Add the fluid base to fill the cup up to the Max Line. Screw the Nutribullet Extractor Blade on to the top of the cup. Invert the cup, press it down into the Nutribullet Power Base and twist it into place. Blast the mixture until it is really smooth (20 or so seconds). **Enjoy!**

Strawberry Heaven

Ingredients

1 Cup/Handful of Mint (40 grams or 1½ oz)
1 Cup/Handful of Green Cabbage (40 grams or 1½ oz)
1 Cup of Blackberries (120 grams or 4 oz)
1 Cup of Strawberries (120 grams or 4 oz)
22 grams or ¾ oz of Flax Seeds
200 ml / 7 fl oz of Water

Protein 8g, Fat 11g, Carb 14g, Fibre 18g, 235 Kcals

Preparation

Place the nuts or seeds into the Tall Cup. Screw the Nutribullet Extractor Blade on to the top of the cup. Invert the cup, press it down into the Nutribullet Power Base and twist it into place. Blast them for 30 seconds. Put the rest of the solid ingredients into the cup and press them down below the Max Line. Add the fluid base to fill the cup up to the Max Line. Screw the Nutribullet Extractor Blade on to the top of the cup. Invert the cup, press it down into the Nutribullet Power Base and twist it into place. Blast the mixture until it is really smooth (20 or so seconds). **Enjoy!**

Watercress and Strawberry Orchard

Ingredients

1 Cup/Handful of Watercress (40 grams or 1½ oz)
1 Cup/Handful of Bok Choy (40 grams or 1½ oz)
1 small Avocado (stoned and peeled) (120 grams or 4 oz)
1 Cup of Strawberries (120 grams or 4 oz)
30 grams or 1 oz of Pecans
200 ml / 7 fl oz of Coconut Milk

Protein 8g, Fat 41g, Carb 16g, Fibre 14g, 487 Kcals

Preparation

Place the nuts or seeds into the Tall Cup. Screw the Nutribullet Extractor Blade on to the top of the cup. Invert the cup, press it down into the Nutribullet Power Base and twist it into place. Blast them for 30 seconds. Put the rest of the solid ingredients into the cup and press them down below the Max Line. Add the fluid base to fill the cup up to the Max Line. Screw the Nutribullet Extractor Blade on to the top of the cup. Invert the cup, press it down into the Nutribullet Power Base and twist it into place. Blast the mixture until it is really smooth (20 or so seconds). **Enjoy!**

Spinach Kiss

Ingredients

1 Cup/Handful of Spinach (40 grams or 1½ oz)
1 Cup/Handful of Rocket/Arugura Lettuce (40 grams or 1½ oz)
1 Cup of Blueberries (120 grams or 4 oz)
1 Cup of Blackberries (120 grams or 4 oz)
30 grams or 1 oz of Walnuts
200 ml / 7 fl oz of Water

Protein 9g, Fat 21g, Carb 23g, Fibre 13g, 331 Kcals

Preparation

Place the nuts or seeds into the Tall Cup. Screw the Nutribullet Extractor Blade on to the top of the cup. Invert the cup, press it down into the Nutribullet Power Base and twist it into place. Blast them for 30 seconds. Put the rest of the solid ingredients into the cup and press them down below the Max Line. Add the fluid base to fill the cup up to the Max Line. Screw the Nutribullet Extractor Blade on to the top of the cup. Invert the cup, press it down into the Nutribullet Power Base and twist it into place. Blast the mixture until it is really smooth (20 or so seconds). **Enjoy!**

Mint embraces Strawberry

Ingredients

2 Cups/Handfuls of Mint (80 grams or 3 oz)
2 Cups of Strawberries (240 grams or 8 oz)
30 grams or 1 oz of Brazil nuts
200 ml / 7 fl oz of Hazelnut Milk

Protein 9g, Fat 25g, Carb 22g, Fibre 13g, 367 Kcals

Preparation

Place the nuts or seeds into the Tall Cup. Screw the Nutribullet Extractor Blade on to the top of the cup. Invert the cup, press it down into the Nutribullet Power Base and twist it into place. Blast them for 30 seconds. Put the rest of the solid ingredients into the cup and press them down below the Max Line. Add the fluid base to fill the cup up to the Max Line. Screw the Nutribullet Extractor Blade on to the top of the cup. Invert the cup, press it down into the Nutribullet Power Base and twist it into place. Blast the mixture until it is really smooth (20 or so seconds). **Enjoy!**

Green Cabbage and Mint Ensemble

Ingredients

1 Cup/Handful of Green Cabbage (40 grams or 1½ oz)
1 Cup/Handful of Mint (40 grams or 1½ oz)
1 small Avocado (stoned and peeled) (120 grams or 4 oz)
1 Cup of Blackberries (120 grams or 4 oz)
22 grams or ¾ oz of Sesame Seeds Hulled
200 ml / 7 fl oz of Almond Milk (Unsweetened)

Protein 11g, Fat 33g, Carb 10g, Fibre 21g, 428 Kcals

Preparation

Place the nuts or seeds into the Tall Cup. Screw the Nutribullet Extractor Blade on to the top of the cup. Invert the cup, press it down into the Nutribullet Power Base and twist it into place. Blast them for 30 seconds. Put the rest of the solid ingredients into the cup and press them down below the Max Line. Add the fluid base to fill the cup up to the Max Line. Screw the Nutribullet Extractor Blade on to the top of the cup. Invert the cup, press it down into the Nutribullet Power Base and twist it into place. Blast the mixture until it is really smooth (20 or so seconds). **Enjoy!**

Cashew Elixir

Ingredients

1 Cup/Handful of Rocket/Arugura Lettuce (40 grams or 1½ oz)
1 Cup/Handful of Watercress (40 grams or 1½ oz)
1 Cup of Strawberries (120 grams or 4 oz)
1 Cup of Blueberries (120 grams or 4 oz)
30 grams or 1 oz of Cashews
200 ml / 7 fl oz of Coconut Milk

Protein 9g, Fat 16g, Carb 36g, Fibre 7g, 323 Kcals

Preparation

Place the nuts or seeds into the Tall Cup. Screw the Nutribullet Extractor Blade on to the top of the cup. Invert the cup, press it down into the Nutribullet Power Base and twist it into place. Blast them for 30 seconds. Put the rest of the solid ingredients into the cup and press them down below the Max Line. Add the fluid base to fill the cup up to the Max Line. Screw the Nutribullet Extractor Blade on to the top of the cup. Invert the cup, press it down into the Nutribullet Power Base and twist it into place. Blast the mixture until it is really smooth (20 or so seconds). **Enjoy!**

Green Cabbage and Bok Choy Panacea

Ingredients

1 Cup/Handful of Green Cabbage (40 grams or 1½ oz)
1 Cup/Handful of Bok Choy (40 grams or 1½ oz)
1 small Avocado (stoned and peeled) (120 grams or 4 oz)
1 Cup of sliced Carrots (120 grams or 4 oz)
30 grams or 1 oz of Almonds
200 ml / 7 fl oz of Hazelnut Milk

Protein 12g, Fat 37g, Carb 20g, Fibre 17g, 491 Kcals

Preparation

Place the nuts or seeds into the Tall Cup. Screw the Nutribullet Extractor Blade on to the top of the cup. Invert the cup, press it down into the Nutribullet Power Base and twist it into place. Blast them for 30 seconds. Put the rest of the solid ingredients into the cup and press them down below the Max Line. Add the fluid base to fill the cup up to the Max Line. Screw the Nutribullet Extractor Blade on to the top of the cup. Invert the cup, press it down into the Nutribullet Power Base and twist it into place. Blast the mixture until it is really smooth (20 or so seconds). **Enjoy!**

Mint goes Rocket

Ingredients

1 Cup/Handful of Mint (40 grams or 1½ oz)
1 Cup/Handful of Rocket/Arugura Lettuce (40 grams or 1½ oz)
1 Cup of Blackberries (120 grams or 4 oz)
1 Cup of sliced Tomato (120 grams or 4 oz)
22 grams or ¾ oz of Flax Seeds
200 ml / 7 fl oz of Coconut Milk

Protein 9g, Fat 12g, Carb 15g, Fibre 17g, 254 Kcals

Preparation

Place the nuts or seeds into the Tall Cup. Screw the Nutribullet Extractor Blade on to the top of the cup. Invert the cup, press it down into the Nutribullet Power Base and twist it into place. Blast them for 30 seconds. Put the rest of the solid ingredients into the cup and press them down below the Max Line. Add the fluid base to fill the cup up to the Max Line. Screw the Nutribullet Extractor Blade on to the top of the cup. Invert the cup, press it down into the Nutribullet Power Base and twist it into place. Blast the mixture until it is really smooth (20 or so seconds). **Enjoy!**

Watercress Galaxy

Ingredients

1 Cup/Handful of Watercress (40 grams or 1½ oz)
1 Cup/Handful of Spinach (40 grams or 1½ oz)
1 Cup of Strawberries (120 grams or 4 oz)
1 Cup of sliced Tomato (120 grams or 4 oz)
22 grams or ¾ oz of Sesame Seeds Hulled
200 ml / 7 fl oz of Water

Protein 8g, Fat 14g, Carb 11g, Fibre 7g, 205 Kcals

Preparation

Place the nuts or seeds into the Tall Cup. Screw the Nutribullet Extractor Blade on to the top of the cup. Invert the cup, press it down into the Nutribullet Power Base and twist it into place. Blast them for 30 seconds. Put the rest of the solid ingredients into the cup and press them down below the Max Line. Add the fluid base to fill the cup up to the Max Line. Screw the Nutribullet Extractor Blade on to the top of the cup. Invert the cup, press it down into the Nutribullet Power Base and twist it into place. Blast the mixture until it is really smooth (20 or so seconds). **Enjoy!**

Blueberry Cornucopia

Ingredients

2 Cups/Handfuls of Rocket/Arugura Lettuce (80 grams or 3 oz)
1 Cup of Blueberries (120 grams or 4 oz)
1 Cup of sliced Carrots (120 grams or 4 oz)
30 grams or 1 oz of Hazelnuts
200 ml / 7 fl oz of Almond Milk (Unsweetened)

Protein 8g, Fat 21g, Carb 26g, Fibre 11g, 343 Kcals

Preparation

Place the nuts or seeds into the Tall Cup. Screw the Nutribullet Extractor Blade on to the top of the cup. Invert the cup, press it down into the Nutribullet Power Base and twist it into place. Blast them for 30 seconds. Put the rest of the solid ingredients into the cup and press them down below the Max Line. Add the fluid base to fill the cup up to the Max Line. Screw the Nutribullet Extractor Blade on to the top of the cup. Invert the cup, press it down into the Nutribullet Power Base and twist it into place. Blast the mixture until it is really smooth (20 or so seconds). **Enjoy!**

Radiant Skin Nourishing Blasts
High in Anti oxidants, Caroteinoids, Polyphenols, Pectin, Zinc, Vitamins A, C

Mint joins Raspberry

Ingredients

1 Cup/Handful of Mint (40 grams or 1½ oz)
1 Cup/Handful of Rocket/Arugura Lettuce (40 grams or 1½ oz)
1 Cup of Raspberries (120 grams or 4 oz)
1 Cup of Prunes (stoned) (120 grams or 4 oz)
22 grams or ¾ oz of Sesame Seeds Hulled
200 ml / 7 fl oz of Dairy Milk Semi Skimmed

Protein 16g, Fat 19g, Carb 22g, Fibre 16g, 322 Kcals

Preparation

Place the nuts or seeds into the Tall Cup. Screw the Nutribullet Extractor Blade on to the top of the cup. Invert the cup, press it down into the Nutribullet Power Base and twist it into place. Blast them for 30 seconds. Put the rest of the solid ingredients into the cup and press them down below the Max Line. Add the fluid base to fill the cup up to the Max Line. Screw the Nutribullet Extractor Blade on to the top of the cup. Invert the cup, press it down into the Nutribullet Power Base and twist it into place. Blast the mixture until it is really smooth (20 or so seconds). **Enjoy!**

Mint and Pumpkin Dictator

Ingredients

2 Cups/Handfuls of Mint (80 grams or 3 oz)
1 Cup of Plum halves (120 grams or 4 oz)
1 Cup of Peach slices (120 grams or 4 oz)
22 grams or ¾ oz of Pumpkin Seeds
200 ml / 7 fl oz of Water

Protein 10g, Fat 11g, Carb 25g, Fibre 10g, 261 Kcals

Preparation

Place the nuts or seeds into the Tall Cup. Screw the Nutribullet Extractor Blade on to the top of the cup. Invert the cup, press it down into the Nutribullet Power Base and twist it into place. Blast them for 30 seconds. Put the rest of the solid ingredients into the cup and press them down below the Max Line. Add the fluid base to fill the cup up to the Max Line. Screw the Nutribullet Extractor Blade on to the top of the cup. Invert the cup, press it down into the Nutribullet Power Base and twist it into place. Blast the mixture until it is really smooth (20 or so seconds). **Enjoy!**

Watercress invites Nectarine

Ingredients

1 Cup/Handful of Watercress (40 grams or 1½ oz)
1 Cup/Handful of Bok Choy (40 grams or 1½ oz)
2 Cups of Nectarine segments (240 grams or 8 oz)
30 grams or 1 oz of Pecans
200 ml / 7 fl oz of Greek Yoghurt

Protein 15g, Fat 41g, Carb 34g, Fibre 8g, 572 Kcals

Preparation

Place the nuts or seeds into the Tall Cup. Screw the Nutribullet Extractor Blade on to the top of the cup. Invert the cup, press it down into the Nutribullet Power Base and twist it into place. Blast them for 30 seconds. Put the rest of the solid ingredients into the cup and press them down below the Max Line. Add the fluid base to fill the cup up to the Max Line. Screw the Nutribullet Extractor Blade on to the top of the cup. Invert the cup, press it down into the Nutribullet Power Base and twist it into place. Blast the mixture until it is really smooth (20 or so seconds). *Enjoy!*

Apple befriends Red Grape

Ingredients

1 Cup/Handful of Green Cabbage (40 grams or 1½ oz)
1 Cup/Handful of Spinach (40 grams or 1½ oz)
1 small Apple (cored) (120 grams or 4 oz)
1 Cup of Red Grapes (120 grams or 4 oz)
30 grams or 1 oz of Cashews
200 ml / 7 fl oz of Water

Protein 8g, Fat 14g, Carb 44g, Fibre 7g, 330 Kcals

Preparation

Place the nuts or seeds into the Tall Cup. Screw the Nutribullet Extractor Blade on to the top of the cup. Invert the cup, press it down into the Nutribullet Power Base and twist it into place. Blast them for 30 seconds. Put the rest of the solid ingredients into the cup and press them down below the Max Line. Add the fluid base to fill the cup up to the Max Line. Screw the Nutribullet Extractor Blade on to the top of the cup. Invert the cup, press it down into the Nutribullet Power Base and twist it into place. Blast the mixture until it is really smooth (20 or so seconds). *Enjoy!*

Rocket Mirage

Ingredients

2 Cups/Handfuls of Rocket/Arugura Lettuce (80 grams or 3 oz)
1 Cup of Strawberries (120 grams or 4 oz)
1 Cup of Nectarine segments (120 grams or 4 oz)
22 grams or ¾ oz of Pumpkin Seeds
200 ml / 7 fl oz of Greek Yoghurt

Protein 17g, Fat 30g, Carb 32g, Fibre 7g, 477 Kcals

Preparation

Place the nuts or seeds into the Tall Cup. Screw the Nutribullet Extractor Blade on to the top of the cup. Invert the cup, press it down into the Nutribullet Power Base and twist it into place. Blast them for 30 seconds. Put the rest of the solid ingredients into the cup and press them down below the Max Line. Add the fluid base to fill the cup up to the Max Line. Screw the Nutribullet Extractor Blade on to the top of the cup. Invert the cup, press it down into the Nutribullet Power Base and twist it into place. Blast the mixture until it is really smooth (20 or so seconds). *Enjoy!*

Watercress and Pecan Embrace

Ingredients

1 Cup/Handful of Watercress (40 grams or 1½ oz)
1 Cup/Handful of Bok Choy (40 grams or 1½ oz)
2 Cups of Raspberries (240 grams or 8 oz)
30 grams or 1 oz of Pecans
200 ml / 7 fl oz of Dairy Milk Semi Skimmed

Protein 14g, Fat 27g, Carb 25g, Fibre 19g, 441 Kcals

Preparation

Place the nuts or seeds into the Tall Cup. Screw the Nutribullet Extractor Blade on to the top of the cup. Invert the cup, press it down into the Nutribullet Power Base and twist it into place. Blast them for 30 seconds. Put the rest of the solid ingredients into the cup and press them down below the Max Line. Add the fluid base to fill the cup up to the Max Line. Screw the Nutribullet Extractor Blade on to the top of the cup. Invert the cup, press it down into the Nutribullet Power Base and twist it into place. Blast the mixture until it is really smooth (20 or so seconds). *Enjoy!*

Cranberry embraces Cashew

Ingredients

1 Cup/Handful of Mint (40 grams or 1½ oz)
1 Cup/Handful of Spinach (40 grams or 1½ oz)
1 Cup of Cranberries (120 grams or 4 oz)
1 small Avocado (stoned and peeled) (120 grams or 4 oz)
30 grams or 1 oz of Cashews
200 ml / 7 fl oz of Water

Protein 11g, Fat 31g, Carb 21g, Fibre 18g, 439 Kcals

Preparation

Place the nuts or seeds into the Tall Cup. Screw the Nutribullet Extractor Blade on to the top of the cup. Invert the cup, press it down into the Nutribullet Power Base and twist it into place. Blast them for 30 seconds. Put the rest of the solid ingredients into the cup and press them down below the Max Line. Add the fluid base to fill the cup up to the Max Line. Screw the Nutribullet Extractor Blade on to the top of the cup. Invert the cup, press it down into the Nutribullet Power Base and twist it into place. Blast the mixture until it is really smooth (20 or so seconds). *Enjoy!*

Green Cabbage and Blackberry Presented

Ingredients

1 Cup/Handful of Rocket/Arugura Lettuce (40 grams or 1½ oz)
1 Cup/Handful of Green Cabbage (40 grams or 1½ oz)
1 Cup of Papaya (120 grams or 4 oz)
1 Cup of Blackberries (120 grams or 4 oz)
22 grams or ¾ oz of Sesame Seeds Hulled
200 ml / 7 fl oz of Dairy Milk Semi Skimmed

Protein 15g, Fat 17g, Carb 28g, Fibre 12g, 350 Kcals

Preparation

Place the nuts or seeds into the Tall Cup. Screw the Nutribullet Extractor Blade on to the top of the cup. Invert the cup, press it down into the Nutribullet Power Base and twist it into place. Blast them for 30 seconds. Put the rest of the solid ingredients into the cup and press them down below the Max Line. Add the fluid base to fill the cup up to the Max Line. Screw the Nutribullet Extractor Blade on to the top of the cup. Invert the cup, press it down into the Nutribullet Power Base and twist it into place. Blast the mixture until it is really smooth (20 or so seconds). *Enjoy!*

Cashew Galaxy

Ingredients

1 Cup/Handful of Bok Choy (40 grams or 1½ oz)
1 Cup/Handful of Rocket/Arugura Lettuce (40 grams or 1½ oz)
½ Cup of Goji Berries Dried (40 grams or 1½ oz)
1 Cup of Guava (120 grams or 4 oz)
30 grams or 1 oz of Cashews
200 ml / 7 fl oz of Greek Yoghurt

Protein 24g, Fat 34g, Carb 54g, Fibre 10g, 637 Kcals

Preparation

Place the nuts or seeds into the Tall Cup. Screw the Nutribullet Extractor Blade on to the top of the cup. Invert the cup, press it down into the Nutribullet Power Base and twist it into place. Blast them for 30 seconds. Put the rest of the solid ingredients into the cup and press them down below the Max Line. Add the fluid base to fill the cup up to the Max Line. Screw the Nutribullet Extractor Blade on to the top of the cup. Invert the cup, press it down into the Nutribullet Power Base and twist it into place. Blast the mixture until it is really smooth (20 or so seconds). **Enjoy!**

Sesame Twist

Ingredients

1 Cup/Handful of Mint (40 grams or 1½ oz)
1 Cup/Handful of Watercress (40 grams or 1½ oz)
1 Cup of Blueberries (120 grams or 4 oz)
1 Cup of Strawberries (120 grams or 4 oz)
22 grams or ¾ oz of Sesame Seeds Hulled
200 ml / 7 fl oz of Water

Protein 8g, Fat 14g, Carb 23g, Fibre 10g, 260 Kcals

Preparation

Place the nuts or seeds into the Tall Cup. Screw the Nutribullet Extractor Blade on to the top of the cup. Invert the cup, press it down into the Nutribullet Power Base and twist it into place. Blast them for 30 seconds. Put the rest of the solid ingredients into the cup and press them down below the Max Line. Add the fluid base to fill the cup up to the Max Line. Screw the Nutribullet Extractor Blade on to the top of the cup. Invert the cup, press it down into the Nutribullet Power Base and twist it into place. Blast the mixture until it is really smooth (20 or so seconds). **Enjoy!**

Goji and Pecan Machine

Ingredients

1 Cup/Handful of Spinach (40 grams or 1½ oz)
1 Cup/Handful of Green Cabbage (40 grams or 1½ oz)
1 Cup of Blueberries (120 grams or 4 oz)
½ Cup of Goji Berries Dried (40 grams or 1½ oz)
30 grams or 1 oz of Pecans
200 ml / 7 fl oz of Greek Yoghurt

Protein 19g, Fat 42g, Carb 51g, Fibre 10g, 673 Kcals

Preparation

Place the nuts or seeds into the Tall Cup. Screw the Nutribullet Extractor Blade on to the top of the cup. Invert the cup, press it down into the Nutribullet Power Base and twist it into place. Blast them for 30 seconds. Put the rest of the solid ingredients into the cup and press them down below the Max Line. Add the fluid base to fill the cup up to the Max Line. Screw the Nutribullet Extractor Blade on to the top of the cup. Invert the cup, press it down into the Nutribullet Power Base and twist it into place. Blast the mixture until it is really smooth (20 or so seconds). **Enjoy!**

Nectarine goes Pumpkin

Ingredients

1 Cup/Handful of Spinach (40 grams or 1½ oz)
1 Cup/Handful of Mint (40 grams or 1½ oz)
1 Cup of Papaya (120 grams or 4 oz)
1 Cup of Nectarine segments (120 grams or 4 oz)
22 grams or ¾ oz of Pumpkin Seeds
200 ml / 7 fl oz of Dairy Milk Semi Skimmed

Protein 17g, Fat 14g, Carb 34g, Fibre 9g, 355 Kcals

Preparation

Place the nuts or seeds into the Tall Cup. Screw the Nutribullet Extractor Blade on to the top of the cup. Invert the cup, press it down into the Nutribullet Power Base and twist it into place. Blast them for 30 seconds. Put the rest of the solid ingredients into the cup and press them down below the Max Line. Add the fluid base to fill the cup up to the Max Line. Screw the Nutribullet Extractor Blade on to the top of the cup. Invert the cup, press it down into the Nutribullet Power Base and twist it into place. Blast the mixture until it is really smooth (20 or so seconds). **Enjoy!**

Watercress hugs Pecan

Ingredients

1 Cup/Handful of Bok Choy (40 grams or 1½ oz)
1 Cup/Handful of Watercress (40 grams or 1½ oz)
1 Cup of Red Grapes (120 grams or 4 oz)
1 Cup of Raspberries (120 grams or 4 oz)
30 grams or 1 oz of Pecans
200 ml / 7 fl oz of Greek Yoghurt

Protein 15g, Fat 42g, Carb 40g, Fibre 12g, 612 Kcals

Preparation

Place the nuts or seeds into the Tall Cup. Screw the Nutribullet Extractor Blade on to the top of the cup. Invert the cup, press it down into the Nutribullet Power Base and twist it into place. Blast them for 30 seconds. Put the rest of the solid ingredients into the cup and press them down below the Max Line. Add the fluid base to fill the cup up to the Max Line. Screw the Nutribullet Extractor Blade on to the top of the cup. Invert the cup, press it down into the Nutribullet Power Base and twist it into place. Blast the mixture until it is really smooth (20 or so seconds). **Enjoy!**

Pumpkin Vision

Ingredients

1 Cup/Handful of Green Cabbage (40 grams or 1½ oz)
1 Cup/Handful of Rocket/Arugura Lettuce (40 grams or 1½ oz)
2 Cups of Plum halves (240 grams or 8 oz)
22 grams or ¾ oz of Pumpkin Seeds
200 ml / 7 fl oz of Dairy Milk Semi Skimmed

Protein 15g, Fat 14g, Carb 38g, Fibre 6g, 350 Kcals

Preparation

Place the nuts or seeds into the Tall Cup. Screw the Nutribullet Extractor Blade on to the top of the cup. Invert the cup, press it down into the Nutribullet Power Base and twist it into place. Blast them for 30 seconds. Put the rest of the solid ingredients into the cup and press them down below the Max Line. Add the fluid base to fill the cup up to the Max Line. Screw the Nutribullet Extractor Blade on to the top of the cup. Invert the cup, press it down into the Nutribullet Power Base and twist it into place. Blast the mixture until it is really smooth (20 or so seconds). **Enjoy!**

Prune Dance

Ingredients

2 Cups/Handfuls of Spinach (80 grams or 3 oz)
1 Cup of Peach slices (120 grams or 4 oz)
1 Cup of Prunes (stoned) (120 grams or 4 oz)
22 grams or ¾ oz of Sesame Seeds Hulled
200 ml / 7 fl oz of Water

Protein 8g, Fat 15g, Carb 15g, Fibre 8g, 201 Kcals

Preparation

Place the nuts or seeds into the Tall Cup. Screw the Nutribullet Extractor Blade on to the top of the cup. Invert the cup, press it down into the Nutribullet Power Base and twist it into place. Blast them for 30 seconds. Put the rest of the solid ingredients into the cup and press them down below the Max Line. Add the fluid base to fill the cup up to the Max Line. Screw the Nutribullet Extractor Blade on to the top of the cup. Invert the cup, press it down into the Nutribullet Power Base and twist it into place. Blast the mixture until it is really smooth (20 or so seconds). *Enjoy!*

Plum in Cashew

Ingredients

2 Cups/Handfuls of Green Cabbage (80 grams or 3 oz)
1 Cup of Guava (120 grams or 4 oz)
1 Cup of Plum halves (120 grams or 4 oz)
30 grams or 1 oz of Cashews
200 ml / 7 fl oz of Dairy Milk Semi Skimmed

Protein 18g, Fat 18g, Carb 43g, Fibre 11g, 422 Kcals

Preparation

Place the nuts or seeds into the Tall Cup. Screw the Nutribullet Extractor Blade on to the top of the cup. Invert the cup, press it down into the Nutribullet Power Base and twist it into place. Blast them for 30 seconds. Put the rest of the solid ingredients into the cup and press them down below the Max Line. Add the fluid base to fill the cup up to the Max Line. Screw the Nutribullet Extractor Blade on to the top of the cup. Invert the cup, press it down into the Nutribullet Power Base and twist it into place. Blast the mixture until it is really smooth (20 or so seconds). *Enjoy!*

Rocket and Watercress Soother

Ingredients

1 Cup/Handful of Rocket/Arugura Lettuce (40 grams or 1½ oz)
1 Cup/Handful of Watercress (40 grams or 1½ oz)
2 Cups of Papaya (240 grams or 8 oz)
22 grams or ¾ oz of Sesame Seeds Hulled
200 ml / 7 fl oz of Greek Yoghurt

Protein 15g, Fat 32g, Carb 34g, Fibre 7g, 495 Kcals

Preparation

Place the nuts or seeds into the Tall Cup. Screw the Nutribullet Extractor Blade on to the top of the cup. Invert the cup, press it down into the Nutribullet Power Base and twist it into place. Blast them for 30 seconds. Put the rest of the solid ingredients into the cup and press them down below the Max Line. Add the fluid base to fill the cup up to the Max Line. Screw the Nutribullet Extractor Blade on to the top of the cup. Invert the cup, press it down into the Nutribullet Power Base and twist it into place. Blast the mixture until it is really smooth (20 or so seconds). *Enjoy!*

Mint kisses Spinach

Ingredients

1 Cup/Handful of Mint (40 grams or 1½ oz)
1 Cup/Handful of Spinach (40 grams or 1½ oz)
1 Cup of Blackberries (120 grams or 4 oz)
1 Cup of Cranberries (120 grams or 4 oz)
30 grams or 1 oz of Cashews
200 ml / 7 fl oz of Water

Protein 10g, Fat 14g, Carb 24g, Fibre 16g, 299 Kcals

Preparation

Place the nuts or seeds into the Tall Cup. Screw the Nutribullet Extractor Blade on to the top of the cup. Invert the cup, press it down into the Nutribullet Power Base and twist it into place. Blast them for 30 seconds. Put the rest of the solid ingredients into the cup and press them down below the Max Line. Add the fluid base to fill the cup up to the Max Line. Screw the Nutribullet Extractor Blade on to the top of the cup. Invert the cup, press it down into the Nutribullet Power Base and twist it into place. Blast the mixture until it is really smooth (20 or so seconds). *Enjoy!*

Bok Choy and Red Grape Blossom

Ingredients

1 Cup/Handful of Bok Choy (40 grams or 1½ oz)
1 Cup/Handful of Green Cabbage (40 grams or 1½ oz)
2 Cups of Red Grapes (240 grams or 8 oz)
22 grams or ¾ oz of Pumpkin Seeds
200 ml / 7 fl oz of Dairy Milk Semi Skimmed

Protein 15g, Fat 14g, Carb 55g, Fibre 5g, 405 Kcals

Preparation

Place the nuts or seeds into the Tall Cup. Screw the Nutribullet Extractor Blade on to the top of the cup. Invert the cup, press it down into the Nutribullet Power Base and twist it into place. Blast them for 30 seconds. Put the rest of the solid ingredients into the cup and press them down below the Max Line. Add the fluid base to fill the cup up to the Max Line. Screw the Nutribullet Extractor Blade on to the top of the cup. Invert the cup, press it down into the Nutribullet Power Base and twist it into place. Blast the mixture until it is really smooth (20 or so seconds). **Enjoy!**

Green Cabbage partners Pecan

Ingredients

1 Cup/Handful of Mint (40 grams or 1½ oz)
1 Cup/Handful of Green Cabbage (40 grams or 1½ oz)
1 small Avocado (stoned and peeled) (120 grams or 4 oz)
1 small Apple (cored) (120 grams or 4 oz)
30 grams or 1 oz of Pecans
200 ml / 7 fl oz of Greek Yoghurt

Protein 16g, Fat 59g, Carb 30g, Fibre 18g, 739 Kcals

Preparation

Place the nuts or seeds into the Tall Cup. Screw the Nutribullet Extractor Blade on to the top of the cup. Invert the cup, press it down into the Nutribullet Power Base and twist it into place. Blast them for 30 seconds. Put the rest of the solid ingredients into the cup and press them down below the Max Line. Add the fluid base to fill the cup up to the Max Line. Screw the Nutribullet Extractor Blade on to the top of the cup. Invert the cup, press it down into the Nutribullet Power Base and twist it into place. Blast the mixture until it is really smooth (20 or so seconds). **Enjoy!**

Immunity Boosting Blasts
Supergreens and foods high in Carotenoids, Sulphoraphane,
Indoles, Fibre, Selenium, Vitamins C, D3, E

Flax Delusion

Ingredients

1 Cup/Handful of Green Cabbage (40 grams or 1½ oz)
1 Cup/Handful of Broccoli Florets (40 grams or 1½ oz)
1 Cup of Blueberries (120 grams or 4 oz)
1 Cup of sliced Tomato (120 grams or 4 oz)
22 grams or ¾ oz of Flax Seeds
200 ml / 7 fl oz of Almond Milk (Unsweetened)

Protein 8g, Fat 12g, Carb 21g, Fibre 13g, 257 Kcals

Preparation

Place the nuts or seeds into the Tall Cup. Screw the Nutribullet Extractor Blade on to the top of the cup. Invert the cup, press it down into the Nutribullet Power Base and twist it into place. Blast them for 30 seconds. Put the rest of the solid ingredients into the cup and press them down below the Max Line. Add the fluid base to fill the cup up to the Max Line. Screw the Nutribullet Extractor Blade on to the top of the cup. Invert the cup, press it down into the Nutribullet Power Base and twist it into place. Blast the mixture until it is really smooth (20 or so seconds). ***Enjoy!***

Spinach and Broccoli Paradox

Ingredients

1 Cup/Handful of Spinach (40 grams or 1½ oz)
1 Cup/Handful of Broccoli Florets (40 grams or 1½ oz)
1 Cup of Tangerine slices (120 grams or 4 oz)
1 Cup of sliced Red Pepper (120 grams or 4 oz)
30 grams or 1 oz of Brazil nuts
200 ml / 7 fl oz of Water

Protein 9g, Fat 21g, Carb 22g, Fibre 9g, 321 Kcals

Preparation

Place the nuts or seeds into the Tall Cup. Screw the Nutribullet Extractor Blade on to the top of the cup. Invert the cup, press it down into the Nutribullet Power Base and twist it into place. Blast them for 30 seconds. Put the rest of the solid ingredients into the cup and press them down below the Max Line. Add the fluid base to fill the cup up to the Max Line. Screw the Nutribullet Extractor Blade on to the top of the cup. Invert the cup, press it down into the Nutribullet Power Base and twist it into place. Blast the mixture until it is really smooth (20 or so seconds). ***Enjoy!***

Green Cabbage and Chia Consortium

Ingredients

2 Cups/Handfuls of Green Cabbage (80 grams or 3 oz)
1 Cup of Red Grapes (120 grams or 4 oz)
1 Cup of sliced Yellow Pepper (120 grams or 4 oz)
22 grams or ¾ oz of Chia Seeds
200 ml / 7 fl oz of Almond Milk (Unsweetened)

Protein 8g, Fat 9g, Carb 30g, Fibre 13g, 268 Kcals

Preparation

Place the nuts or seeds into the Tall Cup. Screw the Nutribullet Extractor Blade on to the top of the cup. Invert the cup, press it down into the Nutribullet Power Base and twist it into place. Blast them for 30 seconds. Put the rest of the solid ingredients into the cup and press them down below the Max Line. Add the fluid base to fill the cup up to the Max Line. Screw the Nutribullet Extractor Blade on to the top of the cup. Invert the cup, press it down into the Nutribullet Power Base and twist it into place. Blast the mixture until it is really smooth (20 or so seconds). *Enjoy!*

Apricot and Carrot Vision

Ingredients

1 Cup/Handful of Spinach (40 grams or 1½ oz)
1 Cup/Handful of Green Cabbage (40 grams or 1½ oz)
1 Cup of Apricot halves (120 grams or 4 oz)
1 Cup of sliced Carrots (120 grams or 4 oz)
22 grams or ¾ oz of Flax Seeds
200 ml / 7 fl oz of Water

Protein 8g, Fat 10g, Carb 21g, Fibre 14g, 243 Kcals

Preparation

Place the nuts or seeds into the Tall Cup. Screw the Nutribullet Extractor Blade on to the top of the cup. Invert the cup, press it down into the Nutribullet Power Base and twist it into place. Blast them for 30 seconds. Put the rest of the solid ingredients into the cup and press them down below the Max Line. Add the fluid base to fill the cup up to the Max Line. Screw the Nutribullet Extractor Blade on to the top of the cup. Invert the cup, press it down into the Nutribullet Power Base and twist it into place. Blast the mixture until it is really smooth (20 or so seconds). *Enjoy!*

Spinach meets Broccoli

Ingredients

1 Cup/Handful of Spinach (40 grams or 1½ oz)
1 Cup/Handful of Broccoli Florets (40 grams or 1½ oz)
1 Cup of Peach slices (120 grams or 4 oz)
1 Cup of diced Beetroot (120 grams or 4 oz)
22 grams or ¾ oz of Chia Seeds
200 ml / 7 fl oz of Almond Milk (Unsweetened)

Protein 10g, Fat 10g, Carb 22g, Fibre 15g, 254 Kcals

Preparation

Place the nuts or seeds into the Tall Cup. Screw the Nutribullet Extractor Blade on to the top of the cup. Invert the cup, press it down into the Nutribullet Power Base and twist it into place. Blast them for 30 seconds. Put the rest of the solid ingredients into the cup and press them down below the Max Line. Add the fluid base to fill the cup up to the Max Line. Screw the Nutribullet Extractor Blade on to the top of the cup. Invert the cup, press it down into the Nutribullet Power Base and twist it into place. Blast the mixture until it is really smooth (20 or so seconds). **Enjoy!**

Strawberry kisses Yellow Pepper

Ingredients

1 Cup/Handful of Green Cabbage (40 grams or 1½ oz)
1 Cup/Handful of Broccoli Florets (40 grams or 1½ oz)
1 Cup of Strawberries (120 grams or 4 oz)
1 Cup of sliced Yellow Pepper (120 grams or 4 oz)
30 grams or 1 oz of Brazil nuts
200 ml / 7 fl oz of Water

Protein 8g, Fat 21g, Carb 16g, Fibre 8g, 292 Kcals

Preparation

Place the nuts or seeds into the Tall Cup. Screw the Nutribullet Extractor Blade on to the top of the cup. Invert the cup, press it down into the Nutribullet Power Base and twist it into place. Blast them for 30 seconds. Put the rest of the solid ingredients into the cup and press them down below the Max Line. Add the fluid base to fill the cup up to the Max Line. Screw the Nutribullet Extractor Blade on to the top of the cup. Invert the cup, press it down into the Nutribullet Power Base and twist it into place. Blast the mixture until it is really smooth (20 or so seconds). **Enjoy!**

Red Pepper Mirage

Ingredients

1 Cup/Handful of Green Cabbage (40 grams or 1½ oz)
1 Cup/Handful of Spinach (40 grams or 1½ oz)
1 Cup of Papaya (120 grams or 4 oz)
1 Cup of sliced Red Pepper (120 grams or 4 oz)
30 grams or 1 oz of Brazil nuts
200 ml / 7 fl oz of Water

Protein 8g, Fat 21g, Carb 19g, Fibre 9g, 305 Kcals

Preparation

Place the nuts or seeds into the Tall Cup. Screw the Nutribullet Extractor Blade on to the top of the cup. Invert the cup, press it down into the Nutribullet Power Base and twist it into place. Blast them for 30 seconds. Put the rest of the solid ingredients into the cup and press them down below the Max Line. Add the fluid base to fill the cup up to the Max Line. Screw the Nutribullet Extractor Blade on to the top of the cup. Invert the cup, press it down into the Nutribullet Power Base and twist it into place. Blast the mixture until it is really smooth (20 or so seconds). **Enjoy!**

Orange embraces Flax

Ingredients

1 Cup/Handful of Broccoli Florets (40 grams or 1½ oz)
1 Cup/Handful of Green Cabbage (40 grams or 1½ oz)
1 Cup of Orange segments (120 grams or 4 oz)
1 Cup of sliced Tomato (120 grams or 4 oz)
22 grams or ¾ oz of Flax Seeds
200 ml / 7 fl oz of Almond Milk (Unsweetened)

Protein 9g, Fat 12g, Carb 18g, Fibre 13g, 245 Kcals

Preparation

Place the nuts or seeds into the Tall Cup. Screw the Nutribullet Extractor Blade on to the top of the cup. Invert the cup, press it down into the Nutribullet Power Base and twist it into place. Blast them for 30 seconds. Put the rest of the solid ingredients into the cup and press them down below the Max Line. Add the fluid base to fill the cup up to the Max Line. Screw the Nutribullet Extractor Blade on to the top of the cup. Invert the cup, press it down into the Nutribullet Power Base and twist it into place. Blast the mixture until it is really smooth (20 or so seconds). **Enjoy!**

Grapefruit and Carrot Salad

Ingredients

1 Cup/Handful of Spinach (40 grams or 1½ oz)
1 Cup/Handful of Green Cabbage (40 grams or 1½ oz)
1 Cup of Grapefruit segments (120 grams or 4 oz)
1 Cup of sliced Carrots (120 grams or 4 oz)
22 grams or ¾ oz of Chia Seeds
200 ml / 7 fl oz of Almond Milk (Unsweetened)

Protein 8g, Fat 10g, Carb 20g, Fibre 15g, 239 Kcals

Preparation

Place the nuts or seeds into the Tall Cup. Screw the Nutribullet Extractor Blade on to the top of the cup. Invert the cup, press it down into the Nutribullet Power Base and twist it into place. Blast them for 30 seconds. Put the rest of the solid ingredients into the cup and press them down below the Max Line. Add the fluid base to fill the cup up to the Max Line. Screw the Nutribullet Extractor Blade on to the top of the cup. Invert the cup, press it down into the Nutribullet Power Base and twist it into place. Blast the mixture until it is really smooth (20 or so seconds). ***Enjoy!***

Mango hugs Flax

Ingredients

1 Cup/Handful of Spinach (40 grams or 1½ oz)
1 Cup/Handful of Broccoli Florets (40 grams or 1½ oz)
1 Cup of Mango slices (120 grams or 4 oz)
1 Cup of diced Beetroot (120 grams or 4 oz)
22 grams or ¾ oz of Flax Seeds
200 ml / 7 fl oz of Water

Protein 9g, Fat 10g, Carb 27g, Fibre 13g, 263 Kcals

Preparation

Place the nuts or seeds into the Tall Cup. Screw the Nutribullet Extractor Blade on to the top of the cup. Invert the cup, press it down into the Nutribullet Power Base and twist it into place. Blast them for 30 seconds. Put the rest of the solid ingredients into the cup and press them down below the Max Line. Add the fluid base to fill the cup up to the Max Line. Screw the Nutribullet Extractor Blade on to the top of the cup. Invert the cup, press it down into the Nutribullet Power Base and twist it into place. Blast the mixture until it is really smooth (20 or so seconds). ***Enjoy!***

Papaya and Red Pepper Sunshine

Ingredients

1 Cup/Handful of Green Cabbage (40 grams or 1½ oz)
1 Cup/Handful of Broccoli Florets (40 grams or 1½ oz)
1 Cup of Papaya (120 grams or 4 oz)
1 Cup of sliced Red Pepper (120 grams or 4 oz)
22 grams or ¾ oz of Chia Seeds
200 ml / 7 fl oz of Almond Milk (Unsweetened)

Protein 8g, Fat 10g, Carb 20g, Fibre 15g, 245 Kcals

Preparation

Place the nuts or seeds into the Tall Cup. Screw the Nutribullet Extractor Blade on to the top of the cup. Invert the cup, press it down into the Nutribullet Power Base and twist it into place. Blast them for 30 seconds. Put the rest of the solid ingredients into the cup and press them down below the Max Line. Add the fluid base to fill the cup up to the Max Line. Screw the Nutribullet Extractor Blade on to the top of the cup. Invert the cup, press it down into the Nutribullet Power Base and twist it into place. Blast the mixture until it is really smooth (20 or so seconds). **Enjoy!**

Green Cabbage Fantasy

Ingredients

1 Cup/Handful of Spinach (40 grams or 1½ oz)
1 Cup/Handful of Green Cabbage (40 grams or 1½ oz)
1 Cup of Peach slices (120 grams or 4 oz)
1 Cup of diced Beetroot (120 grams or 4 oz)
30 grams or 1 oz of Brazil nuts
200 ml / 7 fl oz of Water

Protein 9g, Fat 21g, Carb 21g, Fibre 9g, 315 Kcals

Preparation

Place the nuts or seeds into the Tall Cup. Screw the Nutribullet Extractor Blade on to the top of the cup. Invert the cup, press it down into the Nutribullet Power Base and twist it into place. Blast them for 30 seconds. Put the rest of the solid ingredients into the cup and press them down below the Max Line. Add the fluid base to fill the cup up to the Max Line. Screw the Nutribullet Extractor Blade on to the top of the cup. Invert the cup, press it down into the Nutribullet Power Base and twist it into place. Blast the mixture until it is really smooth (20 or so seconds). **Enjoy!**

Broccoli Delivered

Ingredients

2 Cups/Handfuls of Broccoli Florets (80 grams or 3 oz)
1 Cup of Blueberries (120 grams or 4 oz)
1 Cup of sliced Yellow Pepper (120 grams or 4 oz)
30 grams or 1 oz of Brazil nuts
200 ml / 7 fl oz of Water

Protein 9g, Fat 21g, Carb 24g, Fibre 8g, 325 Kcals

Preparation

Place the nuts or seeds into the Tall Cup. Screw the Nutribullet Extractor Blade on to the top of the cup. Invert the cup, press it down into the Nutribullet Power Base and twist it into place. Blast them for 30 seconds. Put the rest of the solid ingredients into the cup and press them down below the Max Line. Add the fluid base to fill the cup up to the Max Line. Screw the Nutribullet Extractor Blade on to the top of the cup. Invert the cup, press it down into the Nutribullet Power Base and twist it into place. Blast the mixture until it is really smooth (20 or so seconds). ***Enjoy!***

Tangerine Royale

Ingredients

1 Cup/Handful of Spinach (40 grams or 1½ oz)
1 Cup/Handful of Broccoli Florets (40 grams or 1½ oz)
1 Cup of Tangerine slices (120 grams or 4 oz)
1 Cup of sliced Carrots (120 grams or 4 oz)
22 grams or ¾ oz of Chia Seeds
200 ml / 7 fl oz of Almond Milk (Unsweetened)

Protein 9g, Fat 10g, Carb 26g, Fibre 16g, 268 Kcals

Preparation

Place the nuts or seeds into the Tall Cup. Screw the Nutribullet Extractor Blade on to the top of the cup. Invert the cup, press it down into the Nutribullet Power Base and twist it into place. Blast them for 30 seconds. Put the rest of the solid ingredients into the cup and press them down below the Max Line. Add the fluid base to fill the cup up to the Max Line. Screw the Nutribullet Extractor Blade on to the top of the cup. Invert the cup, press it down into the Nutribullet Power Base and twist it into place. Blast the mixture until it is really smooth (20 or so seconds). ***Enjoy!***

Carrot Waterfall

Ingredients

1 Cup/Handful of Spinach (40 grams or 1½ oz)
1 Cup/Handful of Broccoli Florets (40 grams or 1½ oz)
1 Cup of Mango slices (120 grams or 4 oz)
1 Cup of sliced Carrots (120 grams or 4 oz)
22 grams or ¾ oz of Chia Seeds
200 ml / 7 fl oz of Almond Milk (Unsweetened)

Protein 9g, Fat 10g, Carb 28g, Fibre 16g, 276 Kcals

Preparation

Place the nuts or seeds into the Tall Cup. Screw the Nutribullet Extractor Blade on to the top of the cup. Invert the cup, press it down into the Nutribullet Power Base and twist it into place. Blast them for 30 seconds. Put the rest of the solid ingredients into the cup and press them down below the Max Line. Add the fluid base to fill the cup up to the Max Line. Screw the Nutribullet Extractor Blade on to the top of the cup. Invert the cup, press it down into the Nutribullet Power Base and twist it into place. Blast the mixture until it is really smooth (20 or so seconds). **Enjoy!**

Green Cabbage befriends Brazil

Ingredients

1 Cup/Handful of Spinach (40 grams or 1½ oz)
1 Cup/Handful of Green Cabbage (40 grams or 1½ oz)
1 Cup of Strawberries (120 grams or 4 oz)
1 Cup of diced Beetroot (120 grams or 4 oz)
30 grams or 1 oz of Brazil nuts
200 ml / 7 fl oz of Water

Protein 9g, Fat 21g, Carb 18g, Fibre 10g, 306 Kcals

Preparation

Place the nuts or seeds into the Tall Cup. Screw the Nutribullet Extractor Blade on to the top of the cup. Invert the cup, press it down into the Nutribullet Power Base and twist it into place. Blast them for 30 seconds. Put the rest of the solid ingredients into the cup and press them down below the Max Line. Add the fluid base to fill the cup up to the Max Line. Screw the Nutribullet Extractor Blade on to the top of the cup. Invert the cup, press it down into the Nutribullet Power Base and twist it into place. Blast the mixture until it is really smooth (20 or so seconds). **Enjoy!**

Green Cabbage and Spinach Cornucopia

Ingredients

1 Cup/Handful of Green Cabbage (40 grams or 1½ oz)
1 Cup/Handful of Spinach (40 grams or 1½ oz)
1 Cup of Grapefruit segments (120 grams or 4 oz)
1 Cup of sliced Yellow Pepper (120 grams or 4 oz)
22 grams or ¾ oz of Flax Seeds
200 ml / 7 fl oz of Almond Milk (Unsweetened)

Protein 8g, Fat 12g, Carb 16g, Fibre 11g, 233 Kcals

Preparation

Place the nuts or seeds into the Tall Cup. Screw the Nutribullet Extractor Blade on to the top of the cup. Invert the cup, press it down into the Nutribullet Power Base and twist it into place. Blast them for 30 seconds. Put the rest of the solid ingredients into the cup and press them down below the Max Line. Add the fluid base to fill the cup up to the Max Line. Screw the Nutribullet Extractor Blade on to the top of the cup. Invert the cup, press it down into the Nutribullet Power Base and twist it into place. Blast the mixture until it is really smooth (20 or so seconds). **Enjoy!**

Red Grape in Brazil

Ingredients

1 Cup/Handful of Broccoli Florets (40 grams or 1½ oz)
1 Cup/Handful of Spinach (40 grams or 1½ oz)
1 Cup of Red Grapes (120 grams or 4 oz)
1 Cup of sliced Tomato (120 grams or 4 oz)
30 grams or 1 oz of Brazil nuts
200 ml / 7 fl oz of Water

Protein 8g, Fat 21g, Carb 27g, Fibre 7g, 324 Kcals

Preparation

Place the nuts or seeds into the Tall Cup. Screw the Nutribullet Extractor Blade on to the top of the cup. Invert the cup, press it down into the Nutribullet Power Base and twist it into place. Blast them for 30 seconds. Put the rest of the solid ingredients into the cup and press them down below the Max Line. Add the fluid base to fill the cup up to the Max Line. Screw the Nutribullet Extractor Blade on to the top of the cup. Invert the cup, press it down into the Nutribullet Power Base and twist it into place. Blast the mixture until it is really smooth (20 or so seconds). **Enjoy!**

Broccoli joins Apricot

Ingredients

1 Cup/Handful of Broccoli Florets (40 grams or 1½ oz)
1 Cup/Handful of Green Cabbage (40 grams or 1½ oz)
1 Cup of Apricot halves (120 grams or 4 oz)
1 Cup of sliced Red Pepper (120 grams or 4 oz)
22 grams or ¾ oz of Chia Seeds
200 ml / 7 fl oz of Almond Milk (Unsweetened)

Protein 9g, Fat 10g, Carb 20g, Fibre 15g, 251 Kcals

Preparation

Place the nuts or seeds into the Tall Cup. Screw the Nutribullet Extractor Blade on to the top of the cup. Invert the cup, press it down into the Nutribullet Power Base and twist it into place. Blast them for 30 seconds. Put the rest of the solid ingredients into the cup and press them down below the Max Line. Add the fluid base to fill the cup up to the Max Line. Screw the Nutribullet Extractor Blade on to the top of the cup. Invert the cup, press it down into the Nutribullet Power Base and twist it into place. Blast the mixture until it is really smooth (20 or so seconds). **Enjoy!**

Apricot partners Flax

Ingredients

1 Cup/Handful of Spinach (40 grams or 1½ oz)
1 Cup/Handful of Broccoli Florets (40 grams or 1½ oz)
1 Cup of Apricot halves (120 grams or 4 oz)
1 Cup of sliced Yellow Pepper (120 grams or 4 oz)
22 grams or ¾ oz of Flax Seeds
200 ml / 7 fl oz of Almond Milk (Unsweetened)

Protein 10g, Fat 13g, Carb 19g, Fibre 12g, 256 Kcals

Preparation

Place the nuts or seeds into the Tall Cup. Screw the Nutribullet Extractor Blade on to the top of the cup. Invert the cup, press it down into the Nutribullet Power Base and twist it into place. Blast them for 30 seconds. Put the rest of the solid ingredients into the cup and press them down below the Max Line. Add the fluid base to fill the cup up to the Max Line. Screw the Nutribullet Extractor Blade on to the top of the cup. Invert the cup, press it down into the Nutribullet Power Base and twist it into place. Blast the mixture until it is really smooth (20 or so seconds). **Enjoy!**

Immunity Boosting Smoothies
Supergreens and foods high in Carotenoids, Sulphoraphane, Indoles, Fibre, Selenium, Vitamins C, D3, E

Broccoli and Mango Garden

Ingredients

1 Cup/Handful of Broccoli Florets (40 grams or 1½ oz)
1 Cup/Handful of Spinach (40 grams or 1½ oz)
1 Cup of Mango slices (120 grams or 4 oz)
1 Cup of sliced Carrots (120 grams or 4 oz)
200 ml / 7 fl oz of Almond Milk (Unsweetened)

Protein 5g, Fat 3g, Carb 27g, Fibre 8g, 169 Kcals

Preparation

Put all the solid ingredients into the Tall Cup and press them down below the Max Line. Add the fluid base to fill the cup up to the Max Line. Screw the Nutribullet Extractor Blade on to the top of the cup. Invert the cup, press it down into the Nutribullet Power Base and twist it into place. Blast the mixture until it is really smooth (20 or so seconds). *Enjoy!*

Apricot and Beetroot Fiesta

Ingredients

1 Cup/Handful of Green Cabbage (40 grams or 1½ oz)
1 Cup/Handful of Broccoli Florets (40 grams or 1½ oz)
1 Cup of Apricot halves (120 grams or 4 oz)
1 Cup of diced Beetroot (120 grams or 4 oz)
200 ml / 7 fl oz of Water

Protein 5g, Fat 0.9g, Carb 22g, Fibre 8g, 132 Kcals

Preparation

Put all the solid ingredients into the Tall Cup and press them down below the Max Line. Add the fluid base to fill the cup up to the Max Line. Screw the Nutribullet Extractor Blade on to the top of the cup. Invert the cup, press it down into the Nutribullet Power Base and twist it into place. Blast the mixture until it is really smooth (20 or so seconds). *Enjoy!*

Spinach Tango

Ingredients

1 Cup/Handful of Green Cabbage (40 grams or 1½ oz)
1 Cup/Handful of Spinach (40 grams or 1½ oz)
1 Cup of Blueberries (120 grams or 4 oz)
1 Cup of sliced Red Pepper (120 grams or 4 oz)
200 ml / 7 fl oz of Water

Protein 4g, Fat 1.0g, Carb 21g, Fibre 7g, 124 Kcals

Preparation

Put all the solid ingredients into the Tall Cup and press them down below the Max Line. Add the fluid base to fill the cup up to the Max Line. Screw the Nutribullet Extractor Blade on to the top of the cup. Invert the cup, press it down into the Nutribullet Power Base and twist it into place. Blast the mixture until it is really smooth (20 or so seconds). **Enjoy!**

Tangerine and Tomato Mirage

Ingredients

2 Cups/Handfuls of Broccoli Florets (80 grams or 3 oz)
1 Cup of Tangerine slices (120 grams or 4 oz)
1 Cup of sliced Tomato (120 grams or 4 oz)
200 ml / 7 fl oz of Almond Milk (Unsweetened)

Protein 5g, Fat 3g, Carb 21g, Fibre 6g, 138 Kcals

Preparation

Put all the solid ingredients into the Tall Cup and press them down below the Max Line. Add the fluid base to fill the cup up to the Max Line. Screw the Nutribullet Extractor Blade on to the top of the cup. Invert the cup, press it down into the Nutribullet Power Base and twist it into place. Blast the mixture until it is really smooth (20 or so seconds). **Enjoy!**

Spinach partners Broccoli

Ingredients

1 Cup/Handful of Spinach (40 grams or 1½ oz)
1 Cup/Handful of Broccoli Florets (40 grams or 1½ oz)
1 Cup of Red Grapes (120 grams or 4 oz)
1 Cup of sliced Yellow Pepper (120 grams or 4 oz)
200 ml / 7 fl oz of Almond Milk (Unsweetened)

Protein 5g, Fat 3g, Carb 28g, Fibre 5g, 163 Kcals

Preparation

Put all the solid ingredients into the Tall Cup and press them down below the Max Line. Add the fluid base to fill the cup up to the Max Line. Screw the Nutribullet Extractor Blade on to the top of the cup. Invert the cup, press it down into the Nutribullet Power Base and twist it into place. Blast the mixture until it is really smooth (20 or so seconds). *Enjoy!*

Green Cabbage meets Strawberry

Ingredients

1 Cup/Handful of Green Cabbage (40 grams or 1½ oz)
1 Cup/Handful of Broccoli Florets (40 grams or 1½ oz)
1 Cup of Strawberries (120 grams or 4 oz)
1 Cup of sliced Red Pepper (120 grams or 4 oz)
200 ml / 7 fl oz of Water

Protein 4g, Fat 0.9g, Carb 14g, Fibre 7g, 99 Kcals

Preparation

Put all the solid ingredients into the Tall Cup and press them down below the Max Line. Add the fluid base to fill the cup up to the Max Line. Screw the Nutribullet Extractor Blade on to the top of the cup. Invert the cup, press it down into the Nutribullet Power Base and twist it into place. Blast the mixture until it is really smooth (20 or so seconds). *Enjoy!*

Beetroot Bonanza

Ingredients

2 Cups/Handfuls of Spinach (80 grams or 3 oz)
1 Cup of Peach slices (120 grams or 4 oz)
1 Cup of diced Beetroot (120 grams or 4 oz)
200 ml / 7 fl oz of Almond Milk (Unsweetened)

Protein 6g, Fat 3g, Carb 19g, Fibre 8g, 142 Kcals

Preparation

Put all the solid ingredients into the Tall Cup and press them down below the Max Line. Add the fluid base to fill the cup up to the Max Line. Screw the Nutribullet Extractor Blade on to the top of the cup. Invert the cup, press it down into the Nutribullet Power Base and twist it into place. Blast the mixture until it is really smooth (20 or so seconds). **Enjoy!**

Green Cabbage in Orange

Ingredients

1 Cup/Handful of Green Cabbage (40 grams or 1½ oz)
1 Cup/Handful of Spinach (40 grams or 1½ oz)
1 Cup of Orange segments (120 grams or 4 oz)
1 Cup of sliced Carrots (120 grams or 4 oz)
200 ml / 7 fl oz of Water

Protein 4g, Fat 0.6g, Carb 21g, Fibre 8g, 124 Kcals

Preparation

Put all the solid ingredients into the Tall Cup and press them down below the Max Line. Add the fluid base to fill the cup up to the Max Line. Screw the Nutribullet Extractor Blade on to the top of the cup. Invert the cup, press it down into the Nutribullet Power Base and twist it into place. Blast the mixture until it is really smooth (20 or so seconds). **Enjoy!**

Green Cabbage Sonata

Ingredients

1 Cup/Handful of Green Cabbage (40 grams or 1½ oz)
1 Cup/Handful of Broccoli Florets (40 grams or 1½ oz)
1 Cup of Grapefruit segments (120 grams or 4 oz)
1 Cup of sliced Tomato (120 grams or 4 oz)
200 ml / 7 fl oz of Water

Protein 3g, Fat 0.5g, Carb 15g, Fibre 5g, 83 Kcals

Preparation

Put all the solid ingredients into the Tall Cup and press them down below the Max Line. Add the fluid base to fill the cup up to the Max Line. Screw the Nutribullet Extractor Blade on to the top of the cup. Invert the cup, press it down into the Nutribullet Power Base and twist it into place. Blast the mixture until it is really smooth (20 or so seconds). **Enjoy!**

Yellow Pepper Cornucopia

Ingredients

1 Cup/Handful of Spinach (40 grams or 1½ oz)
1 Cup/Handful of Green Cabbage (40 grams or 1½ oz)
1 Cup of Papaya (120 grams or 4 oz)
1 Cup of sliced Yellow Pepper (120 grams or 4 oz)
200 ml / 7 fl oz of Almond Milk (Unsweetened)

Protein 4g, Fat 3g, Carb 18g, Fibre 6g, 129 Kcals

Preparation

Put all the solid ingredients into the Tall Cup and press them down below the Max Line. Add the fluid base to fill the cup up to the Max Line. Screw the Nutribullet Extractor Blade on to the top of the cup. Invert the cup, press it down into the Nutribullet Power Base and twist it into place. Blast the mixture until it is really smooth (20 or so seconds). **Enjoy!**

Apricot and Yellow Pepper Creation

Ingredients

1 Cup/Handful of Spinach (40 grams or 1½ oz)
1 Cup/Handful of Broccoli Florets (40 grams or 1½ oz)
1 Cup of Apricot halves (120 grams or 4 oz)
1 Cup of sliced Yellow Pepper (120 grams or 4 oz)
200 ml / 7 fl oz of Almond Milk (Unsweetened)

Protein 6g, Fat 3g, Carb 19g, Fibre 6g, 138 Kcals

Preparation

Put all the solid ingredients into the Tall Cup and press them down below the Max Line. Add the fluid base to fill the cup up to the Max Line. Screw the Nutribullet Extractor Blade on to the top of the cup. Invert the cup, press it down into the Nutribullet Power Base and twist it into place. Blast the mixture until it is really smooth (20 or so seconds). **Enjoy!**

Spinach and Broccoli Blend

Ingredients

1 Cup/Handful of Spinach (40 grams or 1½ oz)
1 Cup/Handful of Broccoli Florets (40 grams or 1½ oz)
1 Cup of Peach slices (120 grams or 4 oz)
1 Cup of sliced Carrots (120 grams or 4 oz)
200 ml / 7 fl oz of Water

Protein 4g, Fat 0.9g, Carb 20g, Fibre 7g, 118 Kcals

Preparation

Put all the solid ingredients into the Tall Cup and press them down below the Max Line. Add the fluid base to fill the cup up to the Max Line. Screw the Nutribullet Extractor Blade on to the top of the cup. Invert the cup, press it down into the Nutribullet Power Base and twist it into place. Blast the mixture until it is really smooth (20 or so seconds). **Enjoy!**

Spinach and Tangerine Bliss

Ingredients

2 Cups/Handfuls of Spinach (80 grams or 3 oz)
1 Cup of Tangerine slices (120 grams or 4 oz)
1 Cup of diced Beetroot (120 grams or 4 oz)
200 ml / 7 fl oz of Almond Milk (Unsweetened)

Protein 6g, Fat 3g, Carb 23g, Fibre 8g, 159 Kcals

Preparation

Put all the solid ingredients into the Tall Cup and press them down below the Max Line. Add the fluid base to fill the cup up to the Max Line. Screw the Nutribullet Extractor Blade on to the top of the cup. Invert the cup, press it down into the Nutribullet Power Base and twist it into place. Blast the mixture until it is really smooth (20 or so seconds). **Enjoy!**

Broccoli embraces Blueberry

Ingredients

1 Cup/Handful of Green Cabbage (40 grams or 1½ oz)
1 Cup/Handful of Broccoli Florets (40 grams or 1½ oz)
1 Cup of Blueberries (120 grams or 4 oz)
1 Cup of sliced Tomato (120 grams or 4 oz)
200 ml / 7 fl oz of Water

Protein 4g, Fat 0.8g, Carb 21g, Fibre 6g, 113 Kcals

Preparation

Put all the solid ingredients into the Tall Cup and press them down below the Max Line. Add the fluid base to fill the cup up to the Max Line. Screw the Nutribullet Extractor Blade on to the top of the cup. Invert the cup, press it down into the Nutribullet Power Base and twist it into place. Blast the mixture until it is really smooth (20 or so seconds). **Enjoy!**

Papaya Machine

Ingredients

1 Cup/Handful of Spinach (40 grams or 1½ oz)
1 Cup/Handful of Green Cabbage (40 grams or 1½ oz)
1 Cup of Papaya (120 grams or 4 oz)
1 Cup of sliced Red Pepper (120 grams or 4 oz)
200 ml / 7 fl oz of Water

Protein 3g, Fat 0.9g, Carb 18g, Fibre 6g, 107 Kcals

Preparation

Put all the solid ingredients into the Tall Cup and press them down below the Max Line. Add the fluid base to fill the cup up to the Max Line. Screw the Nutribullet Extractor Blade on to the top of the cup. Invert the cup, press it down into the Nutribullet Power Base and twist it into place. Blast the mixture until it is really smooth (20 or so seconds). **Enjoy!**

Carrot Feast

Ingredients

2 Cups/Handfuls of Green Cabbage (80 grams or 3 oz)
1 Cup of Mango slices (120 grams or 4 oz)
1 Cup of sliced Carrots (120 grams or 4 oz)
200 ml / 7 fl oz of Almond Milk (Unsweetened)

Protein 4g, Fat 3g, Carb 27g, Fibre 8g, 167 Kcals

Preparation

Put all the solid ingredients into the Tall Cup and press them down below the Max Line. Add the fluid base to fill the cup up to the Max Line. Screw the Nutribullet Extractor Blade on to the top of the cup. Invert the cup, press it down into the Nutribullet Power Base and twist it into place. Blast the mixture until it is really smooth (20 or so seconds). **Enjoy!**

Green Cabbage and Strawberry Utopia

Ingredients

1 Cup/Handful of Spinach (40 grams or 1½ oz)
1 Cup/Handful of Green Cabbage (40 grams or 1½ oz)
1 Cup of Strawberries (120 grams or 4 oz)
1 Cup of sliced Red Pepper (120 grams or 4 oz)
200 ml / 7 fl oz of Water

Protein 4g, Fat 0.9g, Carb 13g, Fibre 7g, 94 Kcals

Preparation

Put all the solid ingredients into the Tall Cup and press them down below the Max Line. Add the fluid base to fill the cup up to the Max Line. Screw the Nutribullet Extractor Blade on to the top of the cup. Invert the cup, press it down into the Nutribullet Power Base and twist it into place. Blast the mixture until it is really smooth (20 or so seconds). **Enjoy!**

Orange Kiss

Ingredients

1 Cup/Handful of Broccoli Florets (40 grams or 1½ oz)
1 Cup/Handful of Green Cabbage (40 grams or 1½ oz)
1 Cup of Orange segments (120 grams or 4 oz)
1 Cup of diced Beetroot (120 grams or 4 oz)
200 ml / 7 fl oz of Almond Milk (Unsweetened)

Protein 5g, Fat 3g, Carb 22g, Fibre 9g, 157 Kcals

Preparation

Put all the solid ingredients into the Tall Cup and press them down below the Max Line. Add the fluid base to fill the cup up to the Max Line. Screw the Nutribullet Extractor Blade on to the top of the cup. Invert the cup, press it down into the Nutribullet Power Base and twist it into place. Blast the mixture until it is really smooth (20 or so seconds). **Enjoy!**

Apricot Revision

Ingredients

1 Cup/Handful of Spinach (40 grams or 1½ oz)
1 Cup/Handful of Broccoli Florets (40 grams or 1½ oz)
1 Cup of Apricot halves (120 grams or 4 oz)
1 Cup of sliced Red Pepper (120 grams or 4 oz)
200 ml / 7 fl oz of Water

Protein 5g, Fat 1g, Carb 18g, Fibre 7g, 117 Kcals

Preparation

Put all the solid ingredients into the Tall Cup and press them down below the Max Line. Add the fluid base to fill the cup up to the Max Line. Screw the Nutribullet Extractor Blade on to the top of the cup. Invert the cup, press it down into the Nutribullet Power Base and twist it into place. Blast the mixture until it is really smooth (20 or so seconds). **Enjoy!**

Papaya and Carrot Sunrise

Ingredients

2 Cups/Handfuls of Broccoli Florets (80 grams or 3 oz)
1 Cup of Papaya (120 grams or 4 oz)
1 Cup of sliced Carrots (120 grams or 4 oz)
200 ml / 7 fl oz of Almond Milk (Unsweetened)

Protein 5g, Fat 3g, Carb 22g, Fibre 8g, 153 Kcals

Preparation

Put all the solid ingredients into the Tall Cup and press them down below the Max Line. Add the fluid base to fill the cup up to the Max Line. Screw the Nutribullet Extractor Blade on to the top of the cup. Invert the cup, press it down into the Nutribullet Power Base and twist it into place. Blast the mixture until it is really smooth (20 or so seconds). **Enjoy!**

NOTES

CPSIA information can be obtained
at www.ICGtesting.com
Printed in the USA
BVOW04s0850071116
467122BV00009B/77/P